the

10

**Things You
Need** *to* **Eat**

WITHDRAWN

the
10
THINGS YOU
NEED to EAT

And More Than 100 Easy and Delicious Ways to Prepare Them

Dave Lieberman AND Anahad O'Connor

Illustrations by Ronnie Timmons

WM

WILLIAM MORROW

An Imprint of HarperCollinsPublishers

THE 10 THINGS YOU NEED TO EAT. Copyright © 2010 by Dave Lieberman and Anahad O'Connor. All rights reserved. Printed in the United States of America. No part of this book may be used or reproduced in any manner whatsoever without written permission except in the case of brief quotations embodied in critical articles and reviews. For information address HarperCollins Publishers, 10 East 53rd Street, New York, NY 10022.

HarperCollins books may be purchased for educational, business, or sales promotional use. For information please write: Special Markets Department, HarperCollins Publishers, 10 East 53rd Street, New York, NY 10022.

FIRST EDITION

Designed by Jennifer Daddio / Bookmark Design & Media Inc.

Library of Congress Cataloging-in-Publication Data has been applied for.

ISBN 978-0-06-178027-1

10 11 12 13 14   ID4 / RRD   10 9 8 7 6 5 4 3 2

To both our fathers, who ignited our passions for food

CONTENTS

INTRODUCTION

At its core, this book is about the intersection of two polar, opposing forces that every American tries to balance—the desire to eat food that tastes great and the desire to eat food that won't kill you.

In any supermarket, packages slapped with labels announcing zero saturated fat contain foods spiked with artery-clogging trans fats instead. Meals packed with a day's worth of cholesterol and ungodly amounts of sodium are called diet foods because they're low in calories. Cookies loaded with sugar or artificial sweeteners are promoted as low in fat.

The average supermarket is stocked with more than thirty thousand items. But many of us end up making beelines through the aisles to fill our carts with the same grocery list of foods day in and day out. It is all too easy to get stuck with things that are full-flavored but nutrient-devoid. In a sedentary culture that promotes overeating and discourages exercise, these forces drive rates of diabetes, heart disease, and cancer ever higher.

In fact, surveys show that large numbers of Americans are so bombarded with confusing information that they aren't sure exactly what's good for them, so they basically give up, deciding that trying to figure out how to change their eating habits is generally a waste of time.

The sad truth is that sitting in every grocery store in every city across America are basic foods whose health properties are well researched, well documented, and widely accepted—foods that just might extend your expiration date. And yet many of these foods remain underused and underappreciated. Instead we turn to energy bars, health shakes, and other processed foods that clever marketers have dreamed up even though in reality they have few redeeming health benefits.

But it doesn't have to be that way, which is why we wrote this book. What you are about to read is a product of years spent navigating the same health food challenges.

When we met as college roommates a decade ago, our views on food could not have been farther apart. Dave had just returned from a year in Europe, doing some studying, but mostly eating, cooking, and drinking—and it showed. Anahad, on the other hand, was about as lean and lanky as a carrot stick. Anahad arrived at our dorm with beet juice and whole wheat pasta in hand. Dave arrived with cookbooks, German beer mugs, and a couple bottles of Italian wine. Anahad avoided sweets like the plague. Dave held fast to the mantra that if it tastes good, it *is* good.

For a long time, we winced at each other's eating habits, first as buddies at Yale and then as roommates in New York. We seemed to get along everywhere except the kitchen.

As a health writer for the *New York Times*, Anahad was always trying to cut out the things chefs love most, like red meat, bacon, and butter. As a chef, Dave clung to these ingredients tightly and pointed out that Anahad was missing out big-time by subsisting on a diet of raw veggies, naked pastas, and whole grains with no added flavor to liven them up.

Not that this was Anahad's fault. Anyone who tries to eat well knows what a challenge it can be. The foods that Americans tend to associate with satisfaction and deliciousness, like burgers, steaks, and fries, are also the ones that can make us fat and sick. But what if a person wants to eat healthfully without living the life of a culinary monk? Well, that's where things get interesting. And by *interesting* we mean really, really confusing.

Once we started actually considering each other's dietary perspective, we hit on something that united us first in a common frustration and then, ultimately, in a common purpose.

When we started looking for a happy medium between health and good taste, we were dumbfounded by what we encountered. It seems that in this age of conflicting studies, diet fads, and junk foods masquerading as health foods, even people who seek out the healthiest of health foods are left to wonder which ones are really all they're cracked up to be.

The hottest trend in the health food area right now is the rise of so-called superfoods. There is no shortage of superfoods, and you can find dozens upon dozens of them with wonderfully healthful properties. But going around eating a series of unprepared, individual foods is hardly a substitute for sitting down to a proper meal.

To be turned into meals, foods have to be attainable, enjoyable, and easy to work with in the kitchen. But when you take a look at the list of the superfoods trumpeted about these days, how many of them are actually affordable, tasty, *and* easy to incorporate into everyday cooking?

Acai berries, for example, are touted as the latest great thing, but they're expensive and not very versatile. It's not as if you can find a bag of them at your local supermarket to sprinkle some on your morning bowl of oatmeal. Then there's wheatgrass. Walk into any health food store or juice bar in the country and you'll get a sales pitch on its amazing benefits. But have you actually tasted this stuff?! And we've been told a hundred times that cantaloupe is a superfood. But come on. There's precisely one way to eat it, it tastes good only a couple months out of the year, and during the rest of the year it's flavorless and not worth the price.

So while there are many incredibly healthy foods out there, it seems unrealistic to expect that most of them will be incorporated into the average person's daily eating routine.

That's how we came to the conclusion that if we really wanted to help ourselves and others, the focus needed to be on those foods that were incredibly healthy but also affordable, appealing, and versatile in the kitchen. It seemed like such a simple idea, but we didn't really hear anyone else talking about it. And that's when we decided to write this book.

We scoured the superfood landscape, looking for foods that met three criteria: scientifically supported health benefits, extremely easy to find, and so versatile that we could easily build a complete and varied repertoire of home-style, satisfying, and delicious meals around them. Anahad came up with about twenty foods that he felt were scientifically supported as being extraordinarily beneficial to health. He passed this list on, and Dave combed through it with an eye to availability, appeal, and versatility. The list of twenty became ten.

So here you have it: *The 10 Things You Need to Eat: And More Than 100 Easy and Delicious Ways to Prepare Them*. It's the product of a decade-long friendship and a decade-long journey through the American food universe that have turned us both into sticklers for fresh, clean, and responsibly produced food. Today we can proudly say that we share the same food philosophy: Make it good, but make it healthy.

Enjoy!

Dave and Anahad

A NOTE ABOUT SOME
STAPLE INGREDIENTS

Black Pepper

You'll find black pepper in most of the recipes in this book. Since it plays such a central role, it's important to get it right. Always freshly grind your own pepper from whole peppercorns. Never use preground black pepper—in terms of flavor, it's a mere shadow of the freshly ground option.

Canola Oil

The pronounced flavor and lower smoking (burning) temperature of olive oil mean that it's not the perfect oil for all occasions. When we need an oil that's neutral in flavor but still full of heart-healthy fats, we turn to canola oil. Other vegetable oils, such as safflower and sunflower oil, are also good neutral oil options and just as available, but we found evidence that canola oil tops the list in terms of health benefits.

Olive Oil

Given the health benefits of using olive oil as a primary cooking fat, we rely on it heavily throughout the book, not only to sweat vegetables and panfry but also to add a final flavorful flourish to salads and soups. We use solely extra virgin olive oil because it is the most flavorful and purest variety, but we refer to it simply as *olive oil* for the sake of brevity.

Parmesan Cheese

Parmesan pops up again and again in these recipes. There's a good reason for this: First, it's absolutely delicious and makes nearly anything taste better. Second, it's low in fat compared with most other full-flavored cheeses. And last, because it's so flavorful, you don't need to add very much of it to dishes. All this makes it a win-win addition to a healthy cooking repertoire.

Salt

Salt plays an important role in making delicious food, and we call for it in nearly every recipe. You'll find a wide array of salts on the supermarket shelves these days, but when we include salt in a recipe, we're referring to fine sea salt. Never use iodized table salt, because it's too easy to oversalt dishes with it. Occasionally a recipe calls for kosher salt for its coarse grind. Dave has done his best to use salt in moderation, but if you are on a low-sodium diet, simply use salt optionally.

Stocks

Using stocks (chicken, beef, vegetable, and fish broths are all included in these recipes) is a key part of making food that is full-flavored while adding only a negligible amount of fat to your dish. If possible, make your own stocks—it really does make a world of difference in the finished dish. But we know this isn't always realistic for the busy person. If you buy stock, look for low-sodium and organic varieties.

Whole Wheat Flour

White flour makes for creamy, thick sauces and soft, tender baked goods, but these attributes come at the expense of much of the nutrition found in the wheat grains from which the flour is made. The bran and germ of whole wheat grains are rich in fiber and protein along with nutrients such as calcium and iron. But when the grains are refined to make for silky white flour, many of these nutrients are stripped away. That is why we've made a concerted effort to use as much whole wheat flour in place of white flour as possible, while still turning out finished products that are just as delicious and enjoyable as they would have been having only used white flour. Sometimes the results of using just whole wheat flour aren't as favorable, because baked goods can come out tasting heavy or slightly bitter, and in those cases, in the name of taste and enjoyment, the recipes require a minor amount of white flour.

TOMATOES

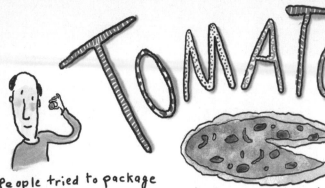

People tried to package all the goodness of tomatoes into a pill form.

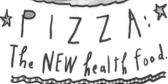

★ PIZZA: ★
The NEW health food.

Because its seeds are on the inside, the tomato is a FRUIT.

Once, people feared tomatoes and NEVER ate them.

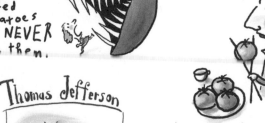

Cooked tomatoes are more nutritious than fresh.

Thomas Jefferson

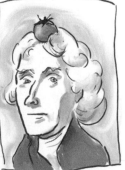

Championed the feared fruit and helped popularize tomatoes.

Today, China produces the most tomatoes.

A very important tip: NEVER, EVER refrigerate a tomato.

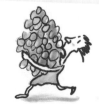

If you plant "determinate" tomatoes, the fruit will ripen all at once.

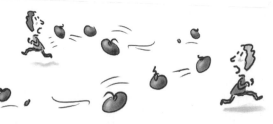

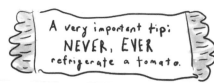

Even today, some still mistakenly avoid tomatoes because they are a member of the Deadly Nightshade family.

1

TOMATOES

Pop quiz: Is pizza junk food?

Ask most Americans, and the answer almost certainly will be yes. How could anything with gobs of cheese and dough *not* be a nutritionist's nightmare? But ask the right scientist, and you may not get the same answer. In fact, not too long ago a team of Italian doctors at a hospital in Milan set out to answer that very question, and what they found might surprise you.

Their objective: to figure out whether eating pizza could play a role in a person's risk of heart disease.

To get their answer, the researchers interviewed and studied about a thousand patients who were hospitalized with various conditions during a four-year period in Milan. Roughly half of those patients were admitted after suffering a heart attack, while the other half showed up with non-heart-related conditions, such as orthopedic disorders.

To be clear, much of what the researchers found was predictable. The heart attack patients were more likely to eat plenty of calories and few fruits and vegetables. They had a history of smoking, hypertension, and diabetes. That's not surprising at all. And they rarely if ever drank alcohol.

But when the scientists looked at pizza consumption, they found something few Americans would ever expect. People who regularly ate pizza—at least one serving a week—were 40 percent less likely to suffer a heart attack than those who never ate it. And frequent eaters—those who had two or more servings a week—were a whopping 60 percent less likely.

Mamma mia!

At this point you might be scratching your head. How is it that an almost universal symbol of junk food could be associated with good health? Well, here's how: Start by throwing out everything you know about American pizza. Then learn about pizza the Italian way. That means going easy on the carbs and bad fats. You won't find the pizza consumed in the Italian study on the menu at your local pizza joint. The Italian pizza had thin crusts and was dressed with olive oil and a moderate amount of cheese—there was no mozzarella jammed into the crusts or piled high in three or four layers.

Second, and most important, in their pizza the Italians loaded up on the sauce, and lots of sauce calls for more tomatoes.

The tomato fruit (yes, a fruit, not a vegetable) has so many remarkable nutrients, like those that contributed to the prevention of heart disease in patients from the Milan study mentioned earlier, that scientists have long sought to extract and bottle them. But to no avail. So far no pill has been able to substitute for the real deal. We'll just have to settle with getting our heart-healthy fix the old-fashioned way by biting into one of those delicious slices of authentic Italian pizza, smothered in marinara sauce.

The amazing thing about tomatoes is that unlike most fruits and vegetables, they practically beg to be cooked, as they are in the pizza sauce, because cooking only enhances their nutritional content. Chopping and heating makes the active compounds in tomatoes more accessible. Even better, mixing in a little healthy fat like olive oil *further* increases your body's ability to absorb those nutrients, because the nutrients are fat-soluble.

In other words, a recipe with plenty of tomatoes—especially cooked—may be just what the doctor ordered.

If that sounds hard to believe, we understand. One study can easily amount to nothing more than a fluke. Replication is the cornerstone of good research. Even an amateur scientist could tell you that. But consider that when a team of researchers led by Howard Sesso at the Harvard School of Public Health studied the diets of nearly forty thousand adult women in 2003, they too uncovered a relationship between tomato consumption and heart disease. They found that women who ate the most tomato sauce and pizza—about ten servings a week—reduced their risk of cardiovascular disease by 30 percent compared with those who ate no more than one and a half servings of tomato-based foods a week.

Still skeptical?

It may help to know that scientists have also looked for a relationship between tomato-based foods and cancer. Take a look at the *International Journal of Cancer* and you'll find a study published in 2003 involving roughly eight thousand people. What the study found was heartening to anyone who appreciates a good Margherita pie. People who ate the most pizza were 59 percent less likely to contract esophageal cancer, 26 percent less likely to develop colon cancer, and 18 percent less likely to contract laryngeal cancer—findings that have been replicated by other researchers.

You don't have to be a mathematician to appreciate those numbers.

Heart disease, cancer . . . so what exactly is the tomato's secret?

For a long time, the idea that it all came down to a compound called *lycopene,* a phytochemical that helps give the tomato its brilliant color, seemed almost undeniable. Lycopene appeared to have unusually strong anticancer and cardiovascular-protective properties, prompting a rush to extract and sell the nutrient in supplement form. But then there was this: while some studies did in fact show that people with high levels of lycopene in their systems gained the coveted benefits, a number of other studies failed to show any link at all. This caused a great deal of confusion. Was it possible that lycopene worked for some people and not for others? Perhaps some people were genetically more susceptible to lycopene's effects, while others were not. Or was it possible that lycopene's reported benefits were just a mirage?

What appears to be the case, we now know, is that lycopene alone is not the answer. The tomato is chock-full of other phytonutrients and vitamins that work in synergy, which is why a number of studies have since shown that eating whole tomato products has a more protective effect than taking lycopene separately. Lycopene may be a powerful nutrient in its own right, but like a general without his army, it is not terribly useful when it goes to battle alone.

But that shouldn't be a problem. The tomato's slight sweetness and mild acidity give it a flavor that has the power to excite. You don't need to be a New Yorker to appreciate a piping-hot, fresh-from-the-oven slice smothered in marinara and fresh mozzarella, and we all know that Italy is as famous for its dishes with tomatoes as it is for its Barolos.

But as odd as it sounds, that wasn't always the case. Before the tomato was loved, it was feared. When European conquistadores first encountered the tomato in South and Central America, they were taken aback by its bright color and strangely alluring appearance, which led them to assume it was poisonous. They were only half right: tomato leaves can be toxic, but obviously the fruit is safe to eat. Still, the conquistadores collected the seeds and took them back to Europe—roughly around the year 1500—thinking the plant would make aesthetically pleasing ornaments. The Latin botanical name used to christen the new fruit is indicative of its dangerous reputation at the time: *Lycopersicon esculentum*, or, in English, "wolfpeach" (the word *tomato* on the other hand was taken from the Nahuatl language spoken by the Aztecs, who named the fruit *tomatl*).

For ages, the tomato was akin to mistletoe: ubiquitous, prized for its beauty, and never to be eaten. Fittingly, it was the Italians who finally broke the taboo and decided to put the tomato to better use as food—and boy, did they ever. It's believed that some of the first Italian recipes featuring the tomato began appearing in the mid-1600s, about a century after the fruit was introduced to Europe. Today almost every dish that Americans recognize as distinctly Italian features the tomato prominently, from spaghetti to lasagne to bruschette and fagioli.

Thanks to the Italians, the idea of the tomato as food spread quickly, and pretty soon the exotic fruit was turning up on dinner tables throughout Europe, Asia, North Africa, and—by the early 1700s—right here in America.

You may have heard recently that one of the first orders of business around the White House for the Obama family was planting a vegetable garden on the South Lawn. Well, they were far from the first presidential family to tend to their own garden. Thomas Jefferson, a lifelong farmer, was said to have cultivated tomatoes perhaps as early as 1781. According to the *Jefferson Encyclopedia*, he recorded planting tomatoes for many years, once writing, "The gardens yield muskmelons, watermelons, tomatas, okra, pomegranates, figs, and the esculent plants of Europe."

Ah, Jefferson—ever the worldly sophisticate. The man who helped bring us democracy and the Declaration obviously knew a great plant when he saw one.

Speaking of sophisticates with a good eye for garden ingredients, Dave likes to point out that one reason the tomato is so tightly woven into the fabric of numerous cultures is its broad range of uses.

Tomatoes are sweet, savory, and acidic all at the same time—a combination that stimulates the palate in a way few other foods can. The Japanese have a name for this quality. They call it umame. It's a characteristic that animal proteins share as well. But tomatoes are one of only a few plants on the planet that possess it.

This unique flavor profile is what makes tomatoes so critical to great-tasting food all over the world. Tomato pulp forms the base for delicious dishes ranging from lamb tagines in Morocco to fish curries in Thailand. And in Italy, of course, the tomato reigns supreme in all forms. Diced fresh tomatoes turn into bruschette; crushed tomatoes turn into pasta sauces; and tomato paste is relied on to give that hallmark depth and complexity to slow-cooked rustic braises up and down the length of the country.

The breadth of what can be done with a tomato is overwhelming, so picking just a dozen recipes to include here was no easy job. As a solution to the maddening task of narrowing the field, I decided to simply include the kind of tomato dishes that I enjoy eating most. Looking back over them now, I realize just how dominant Mediterranean cuisine is in the tomato repertoire. But this is music to Anahad's ears; he often extols the virtues of the Mediterranean diet and the prevalence of long, disease-free life spans in that region. I did, however, manage to squeeze in a delicious Mexico-inspired recipe that turned out to be one of our favorite dishes. And (allow me to indulge for a moment) I tip my hat to my idea of American summer, which for some reason seems to be captured so perfectly in my corn and tomato salad.

When it comes to tomatoes, getting them fresh, locally, and vine-ripened is by far the best way to go. I wait all year for summer to come around so I can gorge on the local New York and New Jersey tomatoes flooding the farmers' markets here in New York City.

The ripe-looking tomatoes available at supermarkets all year are, at best, just a decent substitute for the real local and seasonal thing. These tomatoes often arrive after traveling long distances. To ensure they survive the journey from garden to grocery store, growers often pick them underripe and spray them with ripening agents. This is obviously not ideal, but when you need fresh tomatoes, they're certainly nice to have around.

When fresh tomatoes are out of season, canned tomatoes are often a good alternative. The tomatoes are picked when ripe and subsequently processed to lock in their flavor. And even if I have great summer tomatoes around, I sometimes reach for a can of crushed tomatoes when making a pasta sauce simply because I prefer the flavor of canned tomatoes for certain recipes. On top of that, canned tomatoes are quick and easy, inexpensive, and packed with all the health benefits Anahad mentioned earlier.

So what else is there to say? Head to the market, grab yourself a bag of tomatoes along with a little bit of fresh cheese, and then get ready for our whole wheat pizza, a marinara sauce with some kick, and eight other tip-top tomato recipes that'll have you saying Mangia!

Gazpacho

This wonderfully refreshing cold soup packed with tomatoes and veggies is traditionally served on hot summer days. The only fat in this dish comes in the form of a healthy drizzle of olive oil at the end. SERVES 8

3 ounces soft country bread, any tough crust cut away

2 pounds vine-ripened tomatoes, cored and roughly chopped

½ medium sweet onion, roughly chopped

½ small green bell pepper, roughly chopped

½ English cucumber, roughly chopped (about 1 cup)

1 large garlic clove, finely chopped

3 tablespoons sherry vinegar

½ teaspoon salt

Freshly ground black pepper, plus more for garnish

Olive oil for garnish

Tear the bread into small pieces and put into a large mixing bowl. Cover completely with 1½ cups cold water, pushing all the pieces down so they are completely submerged. Let stand until the bread has soaked up most of the water and is soft enough to fall apart easily, about 10 minutes. Transfer the bread mixture to a food processor along with the remaining ingredients except the olive oil. Process until the mixture is smooth and thick but some texture and flecks of color from the individual ingredients are still visible.

Refrigerate until well chilled before serving, at least 2 hours and up to overnight.

Ladle the mixture into shallow soup bowls and top each serving with a good drizzle of the olive oil and a few more grinds of pepper.

organic tomatoes

Buying organic tomatoes means paying a premium—but is it worth it?

So far, the evidence is mixed. Studies have found that organic produce can have more nutrients than conventionally grown produce. But it all depends on the type of soil, the amount of moisture and irrigation, and even the fruit or vegetable itself. As a result, the final product is not always consistent.

Researchers at the University of California, Davis, for example, found in studies that growing tomatoes organically amplifies their levels of antioxidants. The organic tomatoes in the study had nearly 80 percent higher levels of an antioxidant called quercetin and more than 90 percent higher levels of kaempferol.

But other studies have had less dramatic results, some finding a far smaller difference in nutrient content between organic and conventional tomatoes.

For now you're probably better off sticking to conventional tomatoes unless you don't mind spending the extra money on something that amounts to a roll of the dice.

If you do decide to opt for organic tomatoes and other produce, you can identify them by the numbers on their labels. Organic produce carries a four-digit number beginning with a 9. Conventional produce has a four-digit number that starts with either a 3 or a 4.

Tomato, Black Olive, and Feta Salad

This is essentially a Greek salad without the romaine that many chefs at your local diner throw into the mix. Instead we place all focus on the tomatoes, and, frankly, I don't miss the lettuce one bit. The better the tomatoes, the better the salad, so use the ripest ones you can get your hands on. SERVES 4

3 tablespoons olive oil

3 tablespoons red wine vinegar

I teaspoon dried oregano

Freshly ground black pepper

I pound vine-ripened tomatoes, cut into wedges

½ red onion, halved lengthwise and very thinly sliced crosswise

½ cup pitted, oil-cured black olives

4 ounces of feta cheese, crumbled

Leaves from I small bunch of fresh mint

In a large mixing bowl, whisk together the olive oil, vinegar, oregano, and black pepper to taste. Add the remaining ingredients and toss gently until the tomatoes are coated evenly with dressing.

Divide the salad among 4 salad plates and serve immediately.

OLIVE OIL

The health advantages of incorporating olive oil into your diet are well known and well publicized. In nearly every cooking magazine you browse or cooking show you flip to, you will probably find some reference to extra virgin olive oil. This ancient oil is among the world's greatest sources of monounsaturated fats, which plenty of epidemiological studies have linked to a reduced risk of heart disease, especially when it displaces saturated fats from the diet. These beneficial fats, along with other compounds in olive oil, help keep your arteries healthy and elastic, and they limit the harmful effects of LDL cholesterol (the bad kind).

Here, too, we regard olive oil as one of the great workhorses of the healthy diet. The danger in using olive oil all the time, however, is the risk of its growing tiresome. To avoid this problem we use olive oil in a wide range of applications from the obvious salad dressing and Italian sauce to less obvious dessert recipes.

But because good olive oil has a strong flavor, it is not for every use. Some people use olive oil as their *only* oil. That seems like overkill, akin to using rosemary as your only fresh herb. Instead, rely more heavily on canola oil, which is neutral in flavor and has a high smoking point, which makes it better for high-heat jobs, particularly all kinds of frying. In most cases, reserve olive oil for Mediterranean-inspired dishes or where the grassy, slightly peppery flavor of the olive oil will add a pleasant flavor accent.

Of course, sometimes elevating olive oil's flavor to dominant status is the point. This is the case in a simple, elegant fish *crudo*, finished with nothing more than olive oil, salt, and some lemon juice, or, for example, in the Blueberry, Lemon, and Olive Oil Cake with Smashed Blueberry Sauce on page 236. In those kinds of recipes, it is more than appropriate to celebrate all the flavor nuances of olive oil and relish them with every bite.

Dave's Marinara

Often, the simpler the recipe, the better it tastes. My marinara sauce, with only six ingredients, is so very perfect in its minimalism. This juicy sauce is the best thing to eat with a big bowl of freshly cooked spaghetti. Plus, dinner will be on the table in less than half an hour. What could be better? MAKES ABOUT 1 QUART

¼ cup olive oil

4 large garlic cloves, very finely chopped

One 26-ounce can crushed tomatoes

1 teaspoon dried oregano

1 teaspoon sugar

¼ teaspoon salt

Heat the olive oil in a large skillet over medium-high heat. Add the garlic and cook just until fragrant, no longer than a minute. Add the tomatoes, 1 cup water, oregano, sugar, and salt. Bring the mixture to a simmer, reduce the heat to medium, and simmer for 15 minutes longer.

Broiled Grape Tomatoes over Ricotta

Grape tomatoes are one of the great luxuries of the supermarket. All year you can find sweet, ripe, juicy, firm grape tomatoes at a reasonable price. I enjoy popping them into my mouth like candy, but this appetizer plate brings out the sweetness and intensity of the tomatoes in a special way. Try to find fresh ricotta made by a small producer. This makes a great light meal or a heartier appetizer. Serve with toasted Italian bread rubbed with a cut garlic clove and brushed with olive oil. SERVES 4

I pint grape tomatoes

Kosher salt

About 10 fresh thyme sprigs

2 tablespoons olive oil, plus more for drizzling

2 cups ricotta cheese

Freshly ground black pepper

Preheat the broiler to its highest setting.

Put the grape tomatoes on a foil-lined baking sheet and toss with a generous sprinkle of the kosher salt, the thyme sprigs, and 2 tablespoons of olive oil. Broil about 6 inches from the heat, shaking the pan once or twice, until the tomatoes start to blister and char slightly, about 7 minutes. Remove and set aside to cool slightly.

Set out 4 serving plates and spoon ½ cup ricotta onto each plate; then top each heap of ricotta with roughly an equal number of grape tomatoes. Use the thyme leaves left on the baking sheet to garnish the tomatoes and finish by drizzling each serving with a little olive oil and seasoning generously with pepper.

Blackened Corn and Grape Tomato Salad

Corn and tomatoes are my favorite summer combination, because it captures the essence of the season so well. If you have your grill set up and ready to go anyway, add flavor by grilling the whole ears of corn to blacken them and then just cut off the cooked kernels. Or follow this recipe, which delivers the spirit of the barbecue without the grill.

SERVES 4

---

1 cup fresh corn kernels

Juice of ½ lemon

2 tablespoons mayonnaise

2 tablespoons canola oil

Leaves from about 5 fresh thyme sprigs

Freshly ground black pepper

¼ teaspoon salt

1 pint grape tomatoes, sliced in half lengthwise

½ English cucumber, cut into ½-inch cubes (about 1½ cups)

½ head of radicchio, torn into pieces

1 large shallot, very thinly sliced

Heat a stainless-steel or cast-iron skillet over medium-high heat for about 4 minutes. Add the corn kernels to the pan and toss until blackened evenly, just a couple minutes. Transfer the corn to a plate to cool.

In a large mixing bowl whisk together the lemon juice, mayonnaise, canola oil, thyme leaves, black pepper, and salt. Add the remaining ingredients along with the reserved corn kernels and toss well to coat the salad with the dressing.

tomatoes and prostate cancer

By now, you've probably figured out that it's a great idea to stock up on tomatoes. But if you're a guy, there's even more reason: they may help slash your risk of prostate cancer.

In the United States, prostate cancer is a leading cause of cancer deaths among men. In the year 2008 alone, prostate cancer claimed the lives of an estimated twenty-nine thousand men.

Tomatoes might make a difference for those at risk. Researchers had suspected from years of animal research and various human studies that something in tomatoes may offer protection. So in 2004, scientists at McGill University conducted a meta-analysis that pooled the results of twenty-one human studies on tomatoes and prostate cancer. They found that men who ate the highest levels of raw tomatoes lowered their risk of the disease by 11 percent. But those who ate the most cooked tomatoes slashed their risk twice as much. The reason is that cooking seems to make the nutrients in tomatoes more bioavailable, and adding healthy fats like olive or canola oil increases your body's ability to absorb them.

In other words, whole tomatoes are great, but tomato sauce is even better.

Roasted Garlic and Tomato Soup

This soup is about as simple as it gets. To make sure it wasn't too plain, I added some roasted garlic, at Anahad's request. The result is equally delicious and easy to prepare. SERVES 6

---

2 large heads of garlic

¼ cup olive oil

I medium onion, finely chopped

One 26-ounce can crushed tomatoes

2 bay leaves

I quart chicken or vegetable stock

Salt and freshly ground black pepper

I teaspoon sugar

Preheat the oven to 375°F.

Cut off the very tops of the garlic heads and place the heads on a double layer of aluminum foil. Drizzle 2 tablespoons of the olive oil over the garlic heads and loosely gather the foil around the garlic, leaving the tops exposed. Bake the garlic for about 30 minutes, until soft and the tops start to darken. Set aside to cool.

Heat the remaining 2 tablespoons of olive oil in a 4-quart pot over medium heat. Add the onion and cook, partially covered, until soft and translucent, about 10 minutes. Add the bay leaves, stock, salt and pepper to taste, and the sugar and then squeeze the roasted garlic pulp out of the skins into the soup. Bring the sauce to a simmer, reduce the heat to medium-low, and simmer, partially covered, for another 30 minutes. Remove the bay leaves and use an immersion blender to puree the soup until smooth.

Spicy Tomato, Red Onion, and Pomegranate Jam

Keep a jar of this tomato jam in your refrigerator and you may never have to buy a bottle of ketchup again! It's sweet, tangy, and spicy, and it makes a fantastic accompaniment to cheese, roasted and grilled meats, or anything else your heart desires. Make sure you use "no-sugar" pectin if you want a nice tight set on the jam. MAKES THREE 6-OUNCE JARS

2 pounds plum tomatoes, cored and halved lengthwise

1 medium red onion, halved lengthwise and very thinly sliced lengthwise

1 cup pomegranate juice

1 cup sugar

3 tablespoons red wine vinegar

¼ cup tomato paste

3 star anise pods

2 teaspoons Worcestershire sauce

1 teaspoon hot red pepper flakes

½ teaspoon salt

Combine all of the ingredients in a 4-quart pot and bring the mixture to a simmer over medium heat. Continue to simmer, stirring frequently, until the liquid is almost completely evaporated and is syrupy, about 1 hour and 15 minutes. Remove the star anise and immediately spoon the hot jam into clean preserving jars. Screw on the caps and cool completely and then refrigerate for up to 6 months.

POMEGRANATE

It's no secret anymore that pomegranates are good for you.

There's hardly a supermarket or deli across the country that doesn't stock bottles of POM, the brand that put pomegranates on the health world's radar. According to independent studies, pomegranate has antibacterial properties and may help reduce oxidative stress. It's been shown to be a great source of antioxidants, and research suggests that it may lower the risk of atherosclerosis, or hardening of the arteries.

Even if you love pomegranate juice, drinking mass quantities of it can be a bit of a challenge considering how sweet it is and its very present bitterness.

Fortunately, there are other ways to consume pomegranates. Dave remembers that when he was a kid, whenever his father bought pomegranates, eating them turned into an evening activity. Newspapers were laid out on the kitchen table, spit cups meant for discarded seeds were assembled, bibs were donned, and off they went, tearing through pomegranate after pomegranate. When the dust settled, the walls were splattered with bloodred juice and the kitchen looked like a massacre site.

As much fun as those pomegranate nights were, we couldn't possibly expect normal people to do this, so let's go over some more sane ways of using pomegranates in the kitchen:

- Separate the kernels of the pomegranate and scatter them over salads.
- Serve the pomegranate kernels in a small bowl as part of a cheese plate.
- Make a pomegranate juice sorbet and top each serving of sorbet with fresh pomegranate kernels.

Eggs in Ancho-Tomato Salsa

When was the last time you had eggs for supper? Well, wait no longer for an excuse. This dish is bold enough in flavor and substantial enough to serve on its own as a light meal or as an appetizer before a larger one. Look for ancho chiles that are thick and meaty and make sure you soak them in boiling water for long enough that they are tender before pureeing them into the salsa. SERVES 4 TO 6

I pound plum tomatoes, cored and halved

3 tablespoons canola oil

Boiling water

2 ounces ancho chiles, stems removed

I medium onion, roughly chopped

3 garlic cloves, finely chopped

Juice of I lime

Salt

6 eggs

Leaves from I small bunch of cilantro

Preheat the oven to 400°F.

Place the halved tomatoes on a foil-lined baking sheet and toss with the canola oil to coat well. Roast the tomatoes until they are soft and collapsed, about 25 minutes. Set aside to cool.

Place the chiles in a small mixing bowl and cover with boiling water. Cover the bowl tightly with a piece of plastic wrap. Let stand until the chiles are soft and pliable, about 15 minutes.

When the tomatoes are cool enough to handle, slip off their skins and place them in a food processor along with the softened chiles, onion, garlic, and lime juice. Process until smooth. Season with salt to taste.

Pour the salsa into a large skillet and bring to a simmer over medium heat. Simmer for 10 minutes. Crack one egg at a time into a small bowl and add to the simmering sauce, distributing the eggs evenly throughout the pan. Cover the pan tightly and cook until the egg whites are firm but the yolks are still slightly runny, about 7 minutes.

Remove the eggs from the heat, garnish with the chopped cilantro, and spoon the eggs, along with plenty of sauce onto individual serving plates.

Tomato and Anchovy Braised Artichoke Hearts with Eggplant and Cannellini Beans

Try to find artichokes with longer, heartier stems, which is usually an indication of a good-size heart. After being braised for a couple of hours, they are so creamy and rich I can eat them with a teaspoon and have to remind myself they aren't bad for me. Serve them as the perfect side for any simple Mediterranean-inspired meal. SERVES 6

1½ pounds eggplant, peeled and cut into ½-inch cubes

1½ tablespoons kosher salt

1 lemon

6 large artichokes

One 28-ounce can crushed tomatoes

6 garlic cloves, finely chopped

One 2-ounce can anchovies packed in olive oil, roughly chopped with the oil

½ cup olive oil

One 15-ounce can cannellini beans, rinsed and drained

Freshly grated Parmesan cheese for garnish

Toss the eggplant with the salt in a large mixing bowl. Transfer the eggplant to a fine-mesh sieve and place it over the bowl to collect the liquid. Cover the eggplant with plastic wrap and let stand for 2 hours, tossing it once or twice.

Preheat the oven to 350°F.

Fill a large bowl with water and squeeze half of the lemon into it. Peel as many leaves off the artichokes as possible; then break off the remaining inner leaves, exposing the fuzzy choke. Use a paring knife to cut away the outer layer from the bottoms and stems of the artichokes and use a small spoon to remove the chokes. Immerse the artichokes in the acidulated water as soon as they have been cleaned to prevent them from turning too brown.

Pour the crushed tomatoes into a nonreactive 9 × 13-inch baking dish. Use 1 cup water to loosen any tomato left in the can and pour that into the baking dish as well. Stir the garlic, anchovies, olive oil, and remaining lemon juice into the tomatoes.

Immerse the artichoke hearts in the sauce, covering them as completely as possible. Cover the baking dish very loosely with aluminum foil and bake for 1 hour. Remove from the oven and toss in the cannellini beans and the eggplant. Cover loosely again with the foil and bake for 1 hour longer, until the artichoke hearts are very tender. Garnish with freshly grated Parmesan.

Whole Wheat Triple-Tomato Pizzas

In a cookbook put together by two guys who live in New York City, the city of the Slice, you're bound to get a recipe for pizza. And we aim to deliver! The whole wheat dough works well because it absorbs the moisture of the sauce and the fresh tomatoes. The crust crisps up quite easily even at home-oven temperatures, which are much lower than those of the coal- and wood-fired ovens used by authentic pizzerias.

MAKES FOUR 8-INCH PIZZAS

For the Dough:

2½ cups whole wheat flour

1½ teaspoons salt

1 tablespoon active dry yeast

2 teaspoons sugar

1 cup very warm water (about 110°F)

2 tablespoons olive oil

For the Toppings:

About 1 cup Dave's Marinara
(page 11)

About 16 sun-dried tomatoes packed in olive oil, roughly chopped with the oil

2 cups grated mozzarella cheese

4 large plum tomatoes, cored and thinly sliced

1 teaspoon hot red pepper flakes

1 teaspoon dried basil leaves

Olive oil for drizzling

Freshly grated Parmesan cheese for garnish

Whisk the flour and salt together in a large mixing bowl.

In a separate bowl, combine the yeast, sugar, and warm water and let stand until all the yeast has dissolved and the mixture starts foaming. Add the olive oil and pour the yeast mixture into the flour. Use a fork to combine the two until a loose dough forms.

Transfer the dough to a clean work surface or the bowl of a stand mixer fitted with the dough hook attachment and knead the dough for about 10 minutes. Place the kneaded ball of dough into a large, well-oiled mixing bowl, cover loosely with plastic wrap, and set aside in a warm, draft-free place until the dough has doubled in size, about 1 hour.

Preheat the oven to 400°F.

Place a large baking sheet in the oven (or use two to cook two pizzas at a time) and heat the baking sheet for at least 10 more minutes.

Turn the dough out onto a floured work surface and divide the dough evenly into 4 parts. Roll each part into an even disk, about 8 inches in diameter.

To make a pizza, spread about ¼ cup of the marinara sauce onto a disk of dough, leaving about a ½-inch edge. Scatter a quarter of the sun-dried tomatoes over the sauce, then ½ cup of the mozzarella cheese, followed by some sliced tomatoes, ¼ teaspoon each of the hot red pepper flakes and dried basil, and finally a good drizzle of olive oil.

Use an oven mitt or kitchen towel to remove the hot baking sheet from the oven, place the assembled pizza on it, and return it to the oven to cook for 15 minutes, until the crust is crispy and the cheese is bubbly and golden brown. Garnish the pizza with some freshly grated Parmesan and cut into slices to serve. Repeat for the remaining 3 pizzas.

Linguine with Calamari, Tomatoes, and Green Olives

I imagine old-school fishermen in Naples would throw this dish together for a quick supper. I've kept the sauce fairly simple so you can experience all the individual flavors. It's fresh, tastes like the sea, and is perfect with a bowl of firm linguine. SERVES 6

¼ cup olive oil

¾ cup pitted green olives, roughly chopped

I teaspoon fennel seeds

½ teaspoon hot red pepper flakes

I cup white wine

I teaspoon anchovy paste

One 26-ounce can smooth strained tomatoes

4 garlic cloves, very finely chopped

Salt

I pound linguine

I ½ pounds cleaned whole calamari, tentacles and bodies separated

About 20 fresh basil leaves, roughly chopped

I lemon, cut into 6 wedges, seeds removed

Bring a large pot of water to a boil. Meanwhile, heat the olive oil in a large skillet over medium-high heat. Add the olives, fennel seeds, and hot red pepper flakes and cook just until the spices are fragrant but not browned, no more than a couple minutes. Add the wine, bring to a simmer, and cook until reduced by about half, about 5 minutes. Add the anchovy paste, tomatoes, and garlic and stir well. Return the mixture to a simmer and cook, partially covered, for 15 minutes.

Add some salt to the pot of boiling water and then cook the linguine al dente while you prepare the calamari. Slice the bodies of the calamari into rings about ¼ inch thick and add the rings and the tentacles to the sauce. Continue to simmer until the calamari are just cooked through, about 10 minutes longer.

Season with salt to taste and stir in the basil. Toss the sauce with the drained linguine and serve each portion with a lemon wedge.

AVOCADO

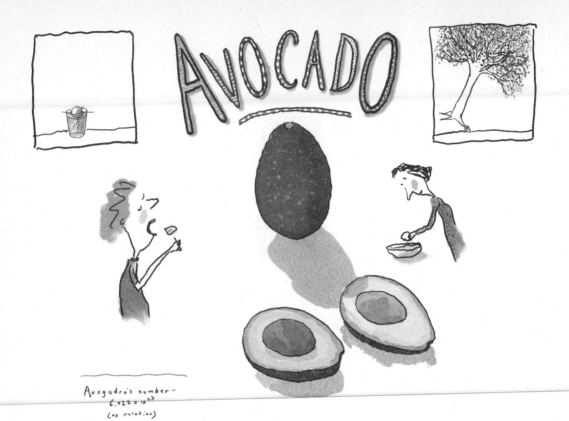

Avogadro's number –
6.022×10^{23}
(no relation)

How to Cut an AVOCADO

1. Slice the fruit lengthwise to the seed.

2. Smack the seed with a knife and pull it out.

3. Slice it in its skin,

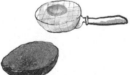

or, just spoon it all out.

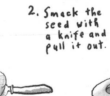

or fill the hole with balsalmic dressing and eat it all before the guests arrive.

2

AVOCADOS

If you're one of those people who still thinks a diet rich in fat will give you heart disease, up your risk of diabetes, and add a foot to your waistline, repeat after us: *fat can be good*.

Most of us have been programmed for years to think that cutting back on fat in every shape and form is the shortest path to better health. But the science could not be any clearer. Focus on the right kind of fat, and you're likely to lose weight, protect your ticker, and lower your risk of all sorts of diseases. Scientists have known this is the case since at least the 1940s, when out of the devastation of World War II came one of the most crucial nutritional discoveries of the last century.

The setting was postwar Europe, southern Greece. In 1947, the Rockefeller Foundation sent researchers and humanitarian aid workers to the palm-dappled island of Crete, a land steeped in ancient history. Previously a paradise, the island had been left in near ruins after a brutal invasion and occupation by German and Italian forces. When the Rockefeller researchers arrived, they were sure they'd find rampant malnutrition. Compared with Americans, the Cretans ate like peasants. Wartime dinner tables were bereft of dairy, and protein was scarce. Instead the locals ate mostly bread, nuts, legumes, some fruits and vegetables, and ample amounts of fat, some from fish and animals and a lot of it from olive oil.

But the diseases that the researchers were sure they'd find among the Cretans were nonexistent. Cardiovascular disease, cancer, and other ills were almost unheard of, and life expectancy was high.

That was in stark contrast to what scientists found when they examined six other countries, especially one much farther north, Finland. Physically, the Finns could not have been more different from the people of Crete. They were loggers and farmers, standing tall, strong, and rugged. Malnutrition was not a concern. Like the Cretans, the Finns ate plenty of fat, most of it from meat, milk, and their national condiment, butter. They also had cholesterol levels that were similar to what was seen in Crete. But unlike the Cretans, the Finns had extraordinary rates of heart disease—the highest in the world. Sharp chest pains were as much a part of reaching midlife in Finland as a fiftieth birthday, except that the chest pains came first. Many Finnish children knew their grandparents only from pictures.

Some researchers thought the difference was genetics, or perhaps Crete's balmy climate. But that theory was quickly disputed: Cretans who migrated to other countries—including tropical ones like Brazil—suffered the same rates of heart disease and cancer as their new countrymen. Speculation soon turned to tobacco. The Finns were known to like their cigarettes. But later studies showed that even in rural areas of Crete where the locals smoked frequently, drank heavily, and had other coronary risk factors, cardiovascular disease was low. Like a Doberman standing sentry over its turf, something in the Cretan diet was fiercely cardio-protective.

We know from more recent studies that the Finns were torturing themselves with the principal fat in their diet, saturated fat, while their Cretan counterparts were reaping huge rewards from the type of fat they were eating, monounsaturated fat.

The benefits of monounsaturated fat cannot be overstated. The medical literature on what it can do for you is enormous. It lowers bad cholesterol, raises the good kind, reduces inflammation, and prevents heart disease. Compared with the artery-gumming effects of saturated fat, it acts like arterial drain cleaner, keeping blood vessels clear and reducing harmful deposits. That's the kind of fat anyone could love.

Balance may be a good thing, but experts say that when it comes to your fat intake, you definitely want the scales to tip heavily in favor of monounsaturated fat. Ask most people where they can find them, however, and beyond a mention of olive or canola oil, you're almost guaranteed a blank stare. So consider yourself a Rockefeller scientist, on the verge of another great discovery. One of nature's most abundant and perhaps surprising sources of monounsaturated gold is a food that plays almost no role in the average person's diet: avocados. If the only time you eat them is in guacamole on Super Bowl Sunday, you're making a huge mistake, like limiting green veggies to St. Paddy's Day.

It's time to make some room in your culinary repertoire.

Ounce for ounce, avocados have more fat than virtually any other fruit, which is why most people typically avoid them, busting them out in the kitchen only a couple times a year for football or Cinco de Mayo. Avocados collect dust on supermarket shelves the rest of the year—making only brief appearances in California rolls and bur-ritos—as we fill our plates with foods that are nutritionally inferior.

Avocados may be high in fat, but the bulk of it is monounsaturated, and like all plant foods they contain no cholesterol. In fact, with their extremely high levels of fiber—about 30 percent of the recommended daily amount in a single cup, the most of any fruit—they actually work to *lower* your cholesterol.

But it gets better. Half an avocado has only 150 calories. That's less than a small order of McDonald's French fries (230 calories), and amazingly, it's even less than a single serving of most Caesar or blue cheese salad dressings (170 to 190 calories), which also come loaded with sodium and both trans and saturated fats. Why dump *that* on a perfectly healthy salad when you can top it off instead with the best fat possible in the form of a few slices of avocado?

If every American made that decision, our health and nutritional landscape would look a lot different. According to a joint report by researchers at the Harvard School of Public Health and Brigham and Women's Hospital in Boston, as many as a hundred thousand cardiac deaths in the United States could be prevented every year if people replaced the bad fats in their diet, particularly trans fats, with monounsaturated fat and its similarly healthy sidekick, nonhydrogenated polyunsaturated fat.

Then there's potassium, the blood-pressure-reducing mineral that bananas are famous for. Bananas are a wonderful food, but avocados contain about 60 percent more potassium. Like carrots in a candy store, avocados rarely get their due.

Consider avocados something of a culinary triple threat: tasty, versatile, and an excellent stand-in for other fats. As a health reporter who's been through the studies and examined the science, I was sold a long time ago. But for all my good intentions, every time I experimented with avocados I would find myself right back in the same place: looking for a bag of blue corn chips.

I just couldn't seem to break out of the guacamole rut.

So I turned to Dave, who had dabbled only occasionally with avocados but quickly came around when he discovered their nutritional profile. In fact, he said, he had been wanting to put them to good use all along.

When I lived in Los Angeles, I thought I had entered an avocado Nirvana, because I had a big, beautiful avocado tree growing right on my deck. It was heavy with fat, green avocados. But I wasn't the only one who had designs on them. Like clockwork, every time the avocados were ready to pick, I'd walk out onto the deck to find that every last one of them was gone, save for a few sad casualties left on the porch that were riddled with little tooth marks. That's when I discovered I had squirrels. So much for my avocado heaven!

That is, until now. Anahad finally gave me another good reason to dream up a bunch of ways to use avocado.

I've always loved avocados, but it wasn't until I finally got around to experimenting with them that I realized just how truly versatile they are. Like most Americans, I've been pretty narrow in my avocado repertoire, sticking to salads, sandwiches, and dips. But as you're about to discover, there's a wide range of uses for avocado, from serving it hot in stews and soups to making it the starting point for delicious smoothies and desserts. Preparing avocado in a sweet way was the most eye-opening part of this exploration for me. But in many parts of the world, particularly in South America and South Asia, enjoying avocado as a dessert with nothing more than some sugar or honey is de rigueur.

Treating avocado as a luscious dessert makes sense, considering its velvety richness. This heart-healthy fat content and mild flavor is exactly what makes avocado such a versatile ingredient. In the following pages, I chop it up finely with crab to create a smooth, creamy dinner that'll leave you saying "Guaca-what?" and then I turn around and puree it with eggs and sugar for some amazing chocolate almond brownies. With endless uses, avocado has everything you need to make it a staple at lunch, dinner, and dessert. Get ready to harness the unlocked potential of a long-overlooked superfood.

Avocado Soup with Cilantro, Coriander, Cumin, and Lime

Whenever I cook with avocados I conjure up the flavors of Mexico, which really works out well, because bright and flavorful ingredients such as lime, cilantro, and spice are just what it takes to bring out the best in creamy avocados. You can serve this soup chilled, but the flavors are much more pronounced and vibrant if you keep it hot. SERVES 8

---

1 large leek

3 tablespoons olive oil

3 medium celery stalks, roughly chopped

1 large onion, roughly chopped

2 bay leaves

1 quart chicken or vegetable stock

½ teaspoon ground coriander

¼ teaspoon ground cumin

1 large ripe Hass avocado, pitted, peeled, and mashed

Juice of 1 lime

Salt and freshly ground black pepper

1 small bunch of scallions, finely chopped

1 small bunch of cilantro, finely chopped

Trim the root end of the leek, cut off the tough green leaves, cut the leek in half lengthwise, and rinse well to remove any grit. Roughly chop the leek.

Heat the olive oil in a large pot or Dutch oven over medium-high heat. Add the leek, celery, and onion and cook for about 5 minutes, or until the vegetables soften. Add the bay leaves, stock, coriander, cumin, avocado, and lime juice and simmer for about 10 minutes. Season with salt and pepper to taste. Ladle into bowls and serve topped with the chopped scallions and cilantro to taste.

avocado varieties

You may notice that these recipes call for Hass avocados. Literally hundreds of varieties of avocados are grown around the world. Most of our avocados come from California, Mexico, or other parts of Central America, where all different kinds are grown for their various sizes, colors, shapes, and flavors.

We love rich, creamy avocados with lots of natural fats that are great for cooking and for your body. Some avocados, such as Florida varieties, tend to have lower fat content and a lighter, even watery taste and consistency. Some people prefer this style of avocado, but the recipes in this book were written with a silky, buttery avocado in mind. The Hass avocado not only consistently fits the bill but also can be found at nearly any supermarket in the country.

When you're shopping for an avocado, you have to stay on your toes if you're going to get one that's perfectly ready. Avocados are picked when they're still hard and take time to soften and ripen. The avocados you'll find at the super-market will be at various stages in the ripening process, so you have to get your hands, and more specifically your fingers, in there.

First, look for avocados with darker skins, because avocado skin darkens as the fruit ripens. Next, pick up your chosen avocado and give it a gentle squeeze. If you can feel any dry crunchy skin or air pockets between the skin and the flesh, you'll have to keep searching. You want the flesh to give slightly to the touch but still have some firm resilience to it. That's the sign of an avocado just asking to be eaten.

Dave's Ultimate Guacamole

No set of avocado recipes would be complete without a recipe for great guacamole. Luckily I have one. My trick is keeping the recipe simple but letting each ingredient really shine through in flavor. I like my guacamole chunky rather than smooth, and I love the way the sweet, juicy tang of some chopped tomato contrasts with the richness of the avocado.

4 large ripe Hass avocados, pitted, peeled, and cut into chunks

Juice of 2 large limes

1 garlic clove, minced

1 small red onion, finely chopped

⅓ cup chopped fresh cilantro leaves

3 plum tomatoes, cored and diced

Salt

Mash the avocados, lime juice, garlic, and red onion together in a large mixing bowl. Stir in the cilantro and tomatoes and season with salt to taste.

Serve immediately or keep covered with a piece of plastic wrap pressed tightly against the surface of the mixture.

what chip to dip

While this guacamole is good enough to eat with anything from vegetable crudités to pita bread, Anahad's favorite way to enjoy guacamole is with a big bowl of baked blue corn chips. Corn chips in general are better for you than flour tortilla chips, and blue corn has slightly greater amounts of antioxidants than yellow or white. Baked chips are a lighter option than the fried version.

ripening avocados—
and keeping them green

As much as we love avocados, they can be a pain. Sometimes they take forever to ripen—as long as six days—and then they can turn bad incredibly fast.

There are all sorts of myths about how to speed up the ripening process. Bury your avocados in a flour bin. Keep them in a bag full of apples. Place them in a brown paper bag and stick them on the windowsill.

But the question is, do any of these tricks work?

Surprisingly, yes. The idea is to keep avocados in a warm, closed environment that allows the gases that ripen them to build up, much the way shutting the windows in a car in the summertime locks in the cold air from the air conditioner. The gas that ripens them is called *ethylene*, and it's released by most plants as they age. But some fruits and vegetables release more than others. Apples and pears release a lot. Berries and cherries release much less.

This is well known in the fruit industry, and it's used to good advantage. Bananas, for example, don't ship very well, so they're usually picked when green, sent to their destinations, and then gassed with ethylene to hasten ripening.

But you don't need a can of ethylene, which is explosive anyway. Just store your avocados somewhere warm and enclosed with a couple of apples or pears the evening before you want to use them. Over the next day or so they should be perfectly ripe and ready to go.

Once an avocado is peeled, the drama is keeping the flesh green. Some people swear by storing guacamole with the avocado pit, for example. But avocados turn brown when an enzyme in them reacts with oxygen. An avocado pit may keep the guacamole it's directly in contact with from browning—simply because it blocks the air—but not the rest of it. A Ping-Pong ball would work exactly the same.

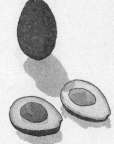

What does work is lemon or lime juice. The acid in the juice slows the reaction between the enzyme and the air. You can also prevent browning with a piece of plastic wrap. Just press it down on the avocado or guacamole to push all the air out, and voilà!

Avocado, Arugula, and Mushroom Salad with Grapefruit Vinaigrette

The spiciness of arugula and the sweet tang of grapefruit in the dressing make great foils for the avocado's rich creaminess. You can toast the pine nuts in a skillet over medium heat or in the oven at 350°F for about seven minutes, but keep a close eye on them, as they can very easily go from brown to burned. SERVES 6

For the Dressing:

Juice of ½ large grapefruit

1 small shallot, minced

1 tablespoon whole-grain mustard

2 tablespoons red wine vinegar

¼ cup extra virgin olive oil

Salt and freshly ground black pepper

For the Salad:

1 large, ripe Hass avocado, pitted, peeled, and thinly sliced

4 ounces baby arugula, preferably wild

4 ounces mushrooms, thinly sliced

¼ cup pine nuts, lightly toasted

1 ounce Parmesan cheese, shaved

To make the dressing, combine all the ingredients in a sealable container and shake vigorously.

To make the salad, combine the avocado, arugula, mushrooms, and pine nuts in a large salad bowl. Toss with the dressing and top with the shaved Parmesan.

Crab and Avocado over Butter Lettuce

Crabmeat is very light and very subtle in flavor, and avocado adds richness without overpowering the crustacean. I like to liven up the combination with lime juice and fresh Thai chile. Quality crabmeat is pretty pricey, so this salad is a good way of making a little crab go a long way.

SERVES 6

---

1 teaspoon whole-grain mustard

Juice of 1 lime

1 large shallot, minced

½ red Thai chile, seeded, deveined, and minced

3 tablespoons minced fresh mint leaves

3 tablespoons minced fresh parsley leaves

3 tablespoons minced fresh cilantro leaves

1 large, ripe Hass avocado, pitted, peeled, and finely diced

8 ounces lump crabmeat

Salt and freshly ground black pepper

1 large head of butter or Bibb lettuce

Olive oil

Whisk the mustard, lime juice, and shallot together in a large mixing bowl. Stir in the chile, mint, parsley, cilantro, avocado, and crabmeat. Season with salt and pepper to taste.

To serve, arrange a couple leaves of lettuce on each plate and top with a spoonful of the crab salad. Drizzle each plate with a little olive oil to finish.

avocado and salad

Salads and fat go together like cookies and milk.

But slather your greens with too much ranch or Caesar and you may as well be using cheese dip. That's why we've created this gut-busting alternative. It's the way to make a healthy salad *even healthier*.

The avocados provide the fat your taste buds are looking for, with heart-healthy results. But the added fat also enhances your body's ability to absorb the nutrients from the other vegetables.

We're not kidding. Scientists at the Ohio State University Comprehensive Cancer Center proved this in 2006. They showed that when groups of people were asked to eat a mixed salad, the people who had avocado added to their salads absorbed two to fifteen times more antioxidants than their peers.

The reason is that some antioxidants are fat-soluble, which means they're poorly absorbed unless there's some fat around. Included in this group are carotenoids, compounds that give many fruits and vegetables their bright colors. More important, studies show they help lower your risk of cancer and other chronic illnesses by eliminating free radicals that roam through your body, tearing at your cells and doing other damage.

That's a lot of science, but it boils down to this: Pair your greens with avocado and you'll be doing yourself a favor. That's more than enough reason to go ahead and whip up this crab and avocado salad.

Avocado Smoothies

Avocados are a wonderful ingredient to use in smoothies. Not only do they add all their heart-healthy properties to the drink, but they also create the creamiest, smoothest smoothies without your having to use any cream or other saturated fats. Because of their mild flavor, they can be mixed with nearly anything, but my personal favorite ingredients are berries, peaches, and bananas. You could also try pineapple, pears, and other fruits—just make sure they're frozen before you put them into the mix.

BERRY BANANA AVOCADO

1 cup frozen blueberries, strawberries, or other berries

1 banana

½ large Hass avocado, pitted and peeled

1 tablespoon honey

¾ cup skim milk, rice milk, or soy milk

Add all the ingredients to a blender and blend until smooth and creamy.

RASPBERRY PEACH AVOCADO

1 cup frozen peach slices

½ cup frozen raspberries

½ large Hass avocado, pitted and peeled

1 tablespoon honey

¾ cup skim milk, rice milk, or soy milk

Add all the ingredients to a blender and blend until smooth and creamy.

Avocado and Spinach Eggs Benedict with Olive Oil "Hollandaise"

Eggs Benedict are big brunch business here in New York City, and you can find nearly everything under the sun stacked on top of an egg and an English muffin. Most of the combinations, loaded with butter and pork fat, will do you no great health favors, but this Benedict sure will. Not only does it combine avocado and spinach, but it also substitutes heart-healthy olive oil for all the butter that normally goes into the Hollandaise sauce. SERVES 4

For the Eggs Benedict:

2 tablespoons canola oil

I small onion, halved and thinly sliced lengthwise

10 ounces frozen chopped spinach, thawed

¼ teaspoon freshly grated nutmeg

Salt and freshly ground black pepper

4 eggs

2 whole wheat English muffins

I ripe Hass avocado, pitted, peeled, and thinly sliced

For the "Hollandaise" Sauce:

½ cup plus 2 tablespoons olive oil

I small shallot, minced

Juice of ½ lemon

I egg yolk

Salt and freshly ground pepper

Heat the canola oil in a large skillet over medium heat. Add the onion and cook, partially covered and stirring often, until softened, about 10 minutes. Add the spinach and season with the nutmeg and salt and pepper to taste. Cook, partially covered, for 5 minutes longer.

To make the "Hollandaise" sauce, heat 2 tablespoons of the olive oil in a small saucepan over medium heat, add the shallot, and cook until softened, about 4 minutes. Remove the pan from the heat, add the lemon juice, and stir in the egg yolk. Reduce the heat to the lowest setting possible and return the pan to the stovetop. Gradually whisk in the remaining ½ cup olive oil until fully incorporated and a rich, thick sauce has formed. Heat just until warm; then remove from the heat. Season with salt and pepper to taste

Fry the eggs sunny side up in a nonstick skillet.

Toast the muffins and top each muffin half with the spinach mixture, avocado, an egg, and some of the "Hollandaise" sauce.

Avocado, Tuna, Tomato, and Cheese Melts

This open-faced sandwich makes a great light meal at any time of day. I recommend some light cheese options here, but you can also play around with more full-bodied and creamier cheeses, like Brie and raclette.

SERVES 4

One 5-ounce can light tuna packed in olive oil

¼ cup olive oil

1 tablespoon minced flat-leaf parsley

1 tablespoon drained capers

1 small shallot, very thinly sliced

Salt and freshly ground black pepper

One 12-inch-long baguette, preferably whole-grain or whole wheat

1 large Hass avocado, pitted, peeled, and thinly sliced

2 large plum or other ripe tomatoes, thinly sliced

Juice of ½ lemon

4 ounces provolone or Swiss cheese, thinly sliced

Position a rack about 10 inches from the broiler element and preheat the broiler to high. Cover a medium baking sheet with aluminum foil and set aside.

To make the tuna mixture, combine the tuna and its oil in a mixing bowl with the olive oil, parsley, capers, and shallot. Season with the salt and pepper to taste.

Slice the baguette in half lengthwise and then into 6-inch lengths. Top each piece with some of the tuna mixture, a few slices of avocado, and some tomato and finish with a squeeze of the lemon juice. Cover with a couple slices of the cheese.

Arrange the open-faced sandwiches on the baking sheet, place under the broiler, and broil until the cheese is melted and bubbly, 5 to 7 minutes.

Avocado and Shrimp Risotto

An avocado risotto is surely not something you come across every day, but it's not as crazy as it sounds. The good fat from the avocado takes the place of the butter that's traditionally used to finish risotto, but the risotto is still creamy and wonderfully flavorful. SERVES 4

---

1 quart seafood or fish stock

3 tablespoons olive oil, plus more to finish

1 large shallot, minced

½ teaspoon hot red pepper flakes

1 cup risotto rice, preferably Carnaroli or Vialone Nano

½ cup dry white wine

2 garlic cloves, pressed or minced

8 ounces shrimp, peeled and deveined

2 Hass avocados, pitted, peeled, and mashed

½ cup finely grated Parmesan cheese, plus more to taste for garnish

Salt and freshly ground pepper

2 tablespoons minced fresh parsley

Bring the stock to a simmer in a medium saucepan over low heat.

Heat the olive oil in a large skillet over medium-low heat. Add the shallot and hot red pepper flakes and cook until translucent, about 5 minutes. Stir in the rice and cook, stirring, until the rice has absorbed a little oil, about 3 minutes. Stir in the wine and cook, stirring, until nearly all the wine has been absorbed. Add the hot stock in 1-cup intervals, stirring constantly until each cup is absorbed. Continue adding the stock until the risotto is creamy and tender; you may need a little more or less than 1 quart of stock (or add in a little hot water as needed). Stir in the garlic, shrimp, and avocados and cook until the shrimp are pink (cooked through), about 5 minutes. Stir in the Parmesan cheese and season with salt and pepper to taste.

Spoon the risotto into 4 bowls and top each serving with a drizzle of olive oil, a pinch more Parmesan, and a couple pinches of parsley.

Chicken, Chile, and Avocado Stew

When I recently traveled to Mexico, I was thrilled by how fresh, ripe avocado was used as a garnish for all sorts of dishes, whether they were hot or cold. I had a terrific spicy chicken soup that was finished with diced avocado. This is my take on it—and it's a great way to make use of those delicious rotisserie chickens that are sold at nearly every super-market these days. SERVES 8

¼ cup olive oil

I large onion, finely chopped

I green bell pepper, finely chopped

I large jalapeño chile, seeded, deveined, and thinly sliced

2 teaspoons chili powder

I teaspoon dried oregano

½ teaspoon ground cumin

One 28-ounce can tomatoes

I quart homemade or low-sodium canned chicken stock

3 garlic cloves, minced

Shredded meat from ½ rotisserie chicken

Salt and freshly ground black pepper

I small bunch of fresh cilantro leaves, roughly chopped

I ripe Hass avocado, pitted, peeled, and roughly chopped

I lime, cut into wedges

Heat the olive oil in a large saucepan or Dutch oven over medium heat. Add the onion, bell pepper, and jalapeño and sauté the vegetables over medium heat until softened, about 10 minutes. Stir in the chili powder, oregano, cumin, tomatoes, stock, and 2 cups water. Bring to a simmer and cook about 1 hour. Add the garlic and chicken and simmer about 30 minutes longer, until the soup has a thick, stewlike consistency. Dish the soup into serving bowls and top each with some cilantro and avocado and a lime wedge.

Chocolate Avocado Mousse

If you've been dying for a guilt-free chocolate mousse, this is your ticket. And it couldn't be simpler. SERVES 6

12 ounces good-quality bittersweet chocolate, chopped

2 teaspoons ground cinnamon

I teaspoon chili powder

I large, ripe Hass avocado, pitted and peeled

¾ cup light brown sugar

6 egg whites

Melt the chocolate with the cinnamon and chili powder in a double boiler over hot water and set aside.

Puree the avocado and brown sugar in a food processor until smooth. With the machine running, pour in the chocolate mixture.

Using a stand mixer or whisk, beat the egg whites until they form soft peaks. Fold the chocolate mixture into the egg whites. Pour the mousse into 6 small serving bowls or wineglasses and refrigerate for at least 1 hour or, covered, overnight.

avocado vs. butter

By now you know that swapping out the bad fat in your desserts and baked treats for the good fat in avocado means better health and less guilt. But it doesn't mean less flavor, which after all is what eating sweets is all about.

You don't have to take our word for it. It's a scientific fact.

In 2008, a team of researchers looked at what happened when they replaced half the butter in a recipe for oatmeal cookies with pureed avocado. They found that compared to the full-butter cookies, the avocado-butter cookies were softer and chewier, and the total fat content plunged by 35 percent, since avocados have less fat per ounce than butter or oil.

Avocado has a similar beneficial effect on cakes and breads—and as you're about to find out, chocolate almond brownies.

Chocolate Almond Avocado Brownies

Really? Avocado brownies? Absolutely! Avocado is so mild in flavor that it is nearly undetectable when paired with lots of brown sugar and chocolate, but it lends its soft creaminess to these rich, chewy brownies. Yum. MAKES 12 LARGE BROWNIES

½ cup whole wheat flour

½ cup Dutch-process cocoa

½ teaspoon salt

I cup almonds

4 ounces good-quality bittersweet chocolate

½ cup canola oil

I large, ripe Hass avocado, pitted and peeled

6 eggs

½ cup granulated sugar

I cup dark brown sugar

Preheat the oven to 350°F. Line a 9 × 13-inch glass baking dish with parchment and grease the parchment.

Whisk the flour, cocoa, and salt together in a large mixing bowl.

Grind the almonds in a food processor until roughly chopped. Stir the nuts into the cocoa mixture.

Break up the chocolate and add the pieces to the food processor. Pulse just until coarsely chopped and stir into the cocoa mixture.

Wipe out the food processor; then add the oil, avocado, eggs, and sugars and process until smooth.

Use a rubber spatula to transfer the avocado mixture to the bowl with the cocoa mixture; then gently fold the dry ingredients into the wet ingredients.

Pour the batter into the baking dish and bake for 35 minutes, until the batter has just barely set in the middle. Allow to cool fully before slicing into 3 × 4-inch brownies.

BEETS

Nature's 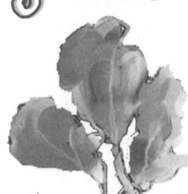 Multivitamin

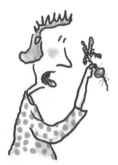

Beets are ugly, until you clean them up →

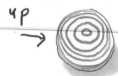

Not everyone likes b e e t s

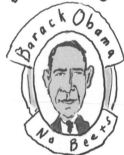

Barack Obama
No Beets

Even though beet greens are a staple in his father's homeland of Kenya, President Obama will not TOUCH THEM.

Aaaaaa Chooooo!

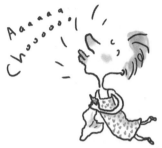

Beets might cure the common cold better than vitamin C.

They're pretty wonderfully good for the heart, too. And BAD for cancer.

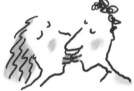

Some have considered beet juice an aphrodisiac.

Their extract can even make dull shoes brilliant.

3

BEETS

If there's one food in the world that could claim the distinction of being nature's multivitamin, the beet might very well be it. Ounce for ounce, the beet, or *Beta vulgaris* as it is known scientifically, boasts what may be a heftier range of nutrients—folate, potassium, iron, fiber, antioxidants, and even a little protein—than virtually any other fruit or vegetable on the planet.

Cultures around the world have been harvesting beets for centuries, many for the plant's medicinal powers. The Romans considered the leaves and roots of the beet a panacea and aphrodisiac.

Even Hippocrates, the father of medicine, was said to have advocated using beet leaves to heal wounds, and if he were alive today, he would surely prescribe many other uses. With the knowledge we have today, he might suggest you stock up on beets to help lower your risk of a range of modern diseases that wreak havoc on the nation's health, from cancer to Alzheimer's and heart disease. Throw away those horse pills you've been taking every morning to get your daily vitamin fix; the beet tops anything you'll find at your local GNC. Plus, we promise, beets are much more delicious and easy to swallow than those oversize capsules.

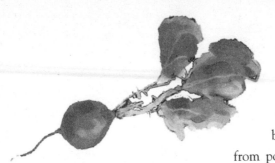

They are hardly easy on the eyes, we admit it. The misshapen roots are usually covered with dirt as if tugged from the soil only minutes before. Shooting from their darkly colored globes are long wispy strands that bring tails to mind. Slightly hairy and far from polished, they are typically stacked far away from their more visually appealing counterparts—the shiny apples, beaming bananas, and plump, red tomatoes that sit front and center in any produce aisle. It is hardly any wonder that beets go overlooked. Even our arugula-loving, Whole Foods–shopping president declared that he steers clear of them!

But for the beet, the role of understudy is undeserved. With the weight of science behind them, beets should play a starring role. As writers, we try to steer clear of clichés, but it's hard to think of another description more befitting the beet than a diamond in the rough.

So how can one beet pack so much punch? For starters, consider the beet's natural pigments, which are not only the source of its strikingly deep crimson color but an indication of just what this superfood is capable of. Besides providing a dose of aesthetic flourish, the beet's pigments are natural antioxidants that fight off free radicals, the harmful molecules that attack the cellular machinery and set in motion processes that can lead to cancer. Studies have shown that these compounds can serve as the bright red stop sign of warning to tumor-inducing molecules.

Among these potent pigments is betalain, the Rodney Dangerfield of antioxidants: it gets no respect. Chances are, you've never felt a cold coming on and thought, "Quick! I've gotta get some betalain." No, the antioxidant that gets all the glory is vitamin C, which cemented its place in medical lore when the Nobel laureate Linus Pauling promoted it decades ago as a cure for common colds and the key to long life. But it may be time to change our way of thinking. Scientists are finding nowadays that betalain can protect the body from the oxidative stress that leads to aging and disease.

Flip through the research and it's hard not to come away impressed. One recent study in the *American Journal of Clinical Nutrition* compared two groups of people, one that was given vitamin C supplements and another that received high doses of betalain in the form of pulp from prickly pears. The group given the betalain had improved antioxidant status, while the vitamin C group showed little difference. Translation: Betalain may be the new vitamin C.

But unlike vitamin C, betalain is not exactly ubiquitous. Only two foods serve as natural sources of it. One is the prickly pear, a fruit that is hard to come by for the average American. The other is the beet, which, fortunately, you can find tucked away in the corner of every produce section in America.

Beets are also brimming with heart-healthy compounds that help lower the risk of cardiovascular disease in several ways. One is by preventing the oxidation of LDL cholesterol. Bear with us for a moment. We know that doesn't sound too impressive, but it will once you understand how critical that can be to the prevention of heart disease.

You're probably already familiar with the notion of two types of cholesterol: the so-called good kind (HDL) and the bad kind (LDL). Well, it turns out that there's a little more to it. Studies have found that LDL cholesterol becomes even more hazardous when it reacts with free radicals—in other words, when it's oxidized. This sets off a terrible chain reaction, sort of like a game of tag. Like the free radicals that maimed it, the newly oxidized LDL *itself* becomes reactive. And as this newly oxidized LDL travels through the body's arteries, it *tags* the lining of the vessels, causing damage that prompts the body to send out inflammatory cells that gather at the site of the damage in an effort to patch up the problem.

But that can cause a traffic jam. Pretty soon a gaggle of cholesterol, platelets, and other cells accumulate at the damaged site, snowballing into a bigger and bigger plaque. Try to picture a traffic accident in the Lincoln Tunnel at rush hour on a Friday afternoon. One bad accident in the middle of the tunnel cuts off the flow of traffic. And that—when it occurs in the wrong arteries—is a recipe for heart disease.

So where do beets come in? Studies have found that some of their phytochemicals help stop the game of tag before it spirals out of control, by helping to prevent LDL molecules from becoming oxidized in the first place.

But you don't have to look to the molecular level to see that beets can make a difference.

One of our favorite studies, and one that really hits home, was carried out in 2008. Because chronic hypertension is a worldwide problem—identified by the World Health Organization in 2002 as a direct cause of 11 percent "of all disease burden"—researchers have long sought simple ways to minimize its toll. With that in mind, a team of

British researchers set out to see if beets could play a role. So they recruited healthy volunteers and then measured their blood pressure and took blood samples after the subjects were given either beet juice or plain old water.

The juice, they concluded, had a marked effect.

"Beetroot juice ingestion lowered blood pressure in healthy volunteers," wrote the scientists, whose results appeared in the journal *Hypertension*, published by the American Heart Association. "There was a lag period of approximately 1 to 2 hours, after ingestion, with a peak drop in blood pressure occurring after 3 to 4 hours."

It's important to point out that the subjects drank 500 ml of beet juice, about the size of a tall glass of juice, or a pint of beer. That's no small amount, and no one is suggesting that you start loading up on cups of pure beet juice. But the take-home message is that it could be a brilliant idea to add some beets to your diet.

And the common cold and cardiovascular disease are not the only areas where the nutrients in beets rise to the challenge. There are just as many studies, if not many more, examining the role that beets may play in lowering the risk of cancer. One way they do this is by ridding the body of the harmful chemicals in processed foods—chief among them nitrates.

Nitrates are the preservatives that manufacturers use to keep sliced turkey, sausages, hot dogs, bacon, and other processed meats from spoiling too quickly, and they can also be found in foods that run the gamut from beer to dried milk. So if they help to keep our food from going bad, what's the problem with them?

Once in the body, nitrates are converted into a carcinogen known as *nitrosamine,* which has been strongly linked to stomach, bladder, and pancreatic cancers. Once on their destructive tear, there is little that can get in their way. But beets are one thing that can stop nitrates dead in their tracks. In various studies scientists have found that beet juice stops the conversion of nitrates to nitrosamine in the stomach, keeping the preservative from taking on its carcinogenic form.

Are you listening, President Obama?

Our president and the first lady may not have made room for beets in their organic White House vegetable garden just yet, but take this as your opportunity to get a leg up on the leader of the free world, at least when it comes to nutrition. Chef Dave has been on to beets long before I started waving studies around and uttering strange words like *betalain.*

I remember one occasion when Dave was asked by Stuart Weitzman, the women's fashion designer, to decorate one of their white satin wedding shoes using only things from his kitchen as part of a fundraiser for the Cancer Research Institute. He went straight for the beets. With rapt curiosity, I watched Dave peel them, cut them into fine dice, boil the heck out of them to extract all of their rosy pigments, and then strain what was left and reduce the dark red liquid to an impossibly crimson dye that made for the most stunningly electric red wedding shoes I had ever seen.

"Those have gotta be the most nutritious wedding shoes ever made," I told him.

While you won't find the recipe for Dave's wedding shoes here, there are lots of other wonderful things to whip up using beets. Dave's love affair with beets, as an ingredient, is clear the minute he starts talking about them:

Beets are the stuff that chefs dream of. Once cooked and peeled, a batch of beets reveals a bright, glistening flesh that promises sweet, earthy flavor and supple texture. Not only do they express a bold, distinctive character in terms of flavor, but they are also a marvel to look at on the plate. Preparing them simply and honestly and arranging them with just a little bit of care can make any chef look like a star. The same goes for a home cook. Beets are so versatile that they are used successfully in everything from soups to desserts. They are equally delicious hot and cold. A fresh beet salad can be just as pleasing as a side of roasted beet—and desserts!

As you're about to see, I take tremendous pride in using beets to make sweet creations. And why not! They are naturally sugary and moist, two of the hallmarks of good baking. They act much like carrots in a carrot cake; hence the recipe for Chocolate Beet Mini-Cakes on page 72. And if intense red-velvet-cake color is what you're looking for, beets will beat out that nasty artificial food coloring any day. Of course, beets more commonly end up in savory dishes, and in this vein there is no end to what can be done with them, from Russian borscht to the classic bistro salad with beets and goat cheese.

With all that in mind, there is only one thing left to say: Grab some fresh beets, a kitchen knife or two, a few pots, and let's go (you too, Mr. President).

Velvety Beet and Leek Soup

I'm kicking off this chapter with Anahad's favorite beet recipe. The first time I made it he couldn't get enough—I think he ate three or four bowls in one sitting. It is pretty darn delicious, I have to say. And it's so simple and beautiful that it can serve as a daily workhorse or brighten up a special dinner party. SERVES 6

¼ cup olive oil

2 large leeks, white and light green parts, thinly sliced

3 celery stalks, thinly sliced

Salt and freshly ground black pepper

8 ounces red beets, peeled and coarsely grated

2 large bay leaves

1 tablespoon whole-grain Dijon mustard

1 quart low-sodium chicken or vegetable stock

½ cup thick Greek-style yogurt

1 small bunch of chives, finely chopped

Heat the olive oil in a 4- to 6-quart pot over medium heat. Add the leeks and the celery and cook until softened, about 7 minutes.

Add salt and pepper to taste, the beets, bay leaves, mustard, and stock. The solids should be covered by a couple of inches of stock; if not, just add some water to raise the level of the liquid. Bring the soup to a simmer and cook until all the vegetables are very tender and the broth is flavorful, about 30 minutes.

Remove the bay leaves, add the yogurt, and puree with an immersion blender until completely smooth. Season again with salt and pepper to taste. Ladle into bowls and garnish with the chopped chives.

cooking beets

There is more than one way to cook a beet. There are many ways in fact!

Boiling is the most common and probably the most traditional way to cook beets. Here's what to do:

First, don't peel the beets! Just put them in a large pot of cold salted water and bring the water to a rolling boil over high heat. Reduce the heat to medium and cook the beets until they are fork-tender. Cooking times will vary depending on the size of the beets, so you may have to remove some of the smaller beets first. Set the cooked beets aside to cool and then simply use your fingers to peel off the skin—it should come off very easily. By leaving the beets unpeeled during the cooking process, you keep the color, flavor, and nutrients from being leached into the water.

Roasting is another favorite cooking method for preparing beets. It is a very streamlined process, and you don't lose any of the flavor or nutrients of the beets:

Preheat the oven to 400°F. Peel the raw beets and cut them to the desired shape and size. Toss the cut beets in some oil and season generously with salt and pepper. Place the seasoned beets on a foil-lined baking sheet, cover loosely with more foil, and roast until the beets are tender, 20 to 45 minutes, depending on size.

Steaming is an oft-overlooked method of cooking beets, but it's a great way to cook them if you're looking to just enjoy them *au naturel*. As with roasting, there's no leaching of flavor, color, or nutrients. To steam beets, peel the raw beets, cut them into the desired shape and size, and place in the top of a steamer. Cover tightly and cook until the beets are tender, 12 to 30 minutes, depending on size.

Beet Juice Drinks

All of these drinks operate on the same concept: push a bunch of fresh fruits and vegetables through a good juicer, stir, and serve. I've listed the amount of juice of each type that you need rather than the weight or quantity of each ingredient because every batch of fruits and veggies will yield different amounts of juice. Juicing is the only way I know to realistically consume this much produce, and that's what makes these juices so darn healthy. As an added benefit, they're also delicious.

ALL JUICE RECIPES MAKE 8-OUNCE SERVINGS

BEET APPLE GINGER JUICE

¾ cup fresh beet juice

1 cup fresh apple juice

2 tablespoons fresh ginger juice

Stir the juices together and serve.

BEET PEAR GRAPEFRUIT JUICE

1 cup fresh pear juice

¾ cup fresh beet juice

½ cup fresh grapefruit juice

Stir the juices together and serve.

BEET CARROT ORANGE JUICE

1 cup fresh carrot juice

¾ cup fresh beet juice

½ cup fresh orange juice

Stir the juices together and serve.

BEET BANANA MANGO SMOOTHIE

¾ cup fresh beet juice

1 banana, peeled

1 mango, peeled and pitted

Ice

Combine the beet juice and fruits in a blender, add a couple handfuls of ice, and blend until smooth.

Beet and Avocado "Tartare" over Smoked Salmon

I love fish tartare most of all for its silky consistency. This beet tartare has the same silkiness from the ripe avocado that I've thrown into the mix. The smokiness added by the salmon makes for a nice extra element of flavor. SERVES 6

1 small shallot, minced

1 tablespoon whole-grain mustard

¼ cup red wine vinegar

¼ cup olive oil, plus more for drizzling

Salt and freshly ground black pepper

Leaves from 1 small bunch of fresh thyme

12 ounces golden beets, boiled, peeled (see page 55), and cut into ¼-inch cubes

1 ripe Haas avocado, pitted, peeled, and finely diced

12 ounces sliced smoked salmon

4 ounces soft goat cheese

⅓ cup finely chopped toasted pecans

To make the dressing, whisk the shallot, mustard, vinegar, olive oil, salt and pepper to taste, and half of the thyme together in a medium bowl. Add the beets, toss them in the dressing, and let stand at room temperature or covered in the fridge overnight or for at least 30 minutes. Drain the liquid from the beets, add the avocado, and mix gently.

To serve, divide the smoked salmon slices among 6 salad plates, top the salmon with a mound of the beet and avocado "tartare," crumble on a bit of goat cheese, and scatter pecans over the top. Finish each with a drizzle of the olive oil and a pinch or two of the remaining thyme.

is juicing all it's cracked up to be?

The juice craze of the late eighties and early nineties—when hypercaffeinated TV pitchmen hawked countertop juicers that held the cure to everything from baldness to cancer and even impotence—is long gone. Many of those claims, backed by little or no science, were more romance than reality.

But infomercials notwithstanding, there is still plenty of reason to fire up the juicer on a regular basis.

More recent research suggests that juicing releases vitamins and nutrients from plant cells (without the heat damage that can be caused by cooking), increasing their bioavailability and allowing them to be absorbed more easily. You can also pack many more servings of fruits and vegetables into a cup than you can eat off a plate.

True, the juicing process does remove some fibrous material. But the upside to adding fresh juice to your weekly diet is compelling.

One study in 2006 that followed two thousand Americans for a decade found that those who drank at least 3 cups of fruit or vegetable juice a week had a 76 percent lower risk of developing Alzheimer's disease later on than those who had less than one a week, possibly because of the high concentration of polyphenols in fresh juice.

Others have found that people who add juice to their diets absorb greater amounts of certain nutrients—like lutein and alpha-carotene—than those who consume their vegetables only in cooked or raw form.

Jam-Packed Juicing Muffins

When Anahad and I were experimenting with our juice recipes, we were left with tons of fibrous pulp in the juicer's "waste" basket. During cleanup one day, Anahad scooped up a handful of pulp. He shook his head and said, "This is all fiber—what a shame to just throw it all away. Isn't there a way to put this to use?" These muffins are my answer. They're moist, satisfying, and absolutely delicious.   MAKES 24 MUFFINS

1¾ cups juicing pulp

½ cup good-quality orange juice

½ cup thick Greek-style yogurt

4 eggs

¾ cup canola oil

1 teaspoon vanilla extract

3 tablespoons honey

¾ cup sugar

1½ cups whole wheat flour

1 teaspoon baking powder

1 teaspoon baking soda

½ teaspoon fine salt

½ cup raisins

Preheat the oven to 350°F and oil a 24-muffin tin.

In a large bowl, combine the pulp, juice, yogurt, eggs, oil, vanilla extract, honey, and sugar and whisk thoroughly.

In a separate bowl, combine the flour, baking powder, baking soda, and salt and whisk thoroughly.

Fold the dry ingredients into the wet mixture and mix until just combined. Do not overmix, or the muffins will be tough. Fold in the raisins.

Fill the muffin cups about three-quarters full with batter. Bake for 25 minutes, or until a toothpick inserted into the center of a muffin comes out clean and the muffins start to pull away from the sides of the pan. Cool before serving.

Beet, Apple, Carrot, and Walnut Salad

This salad is vibrant, sweet, tart, and crunchy. Where else can you find a sweet side dish that isn't loaded with unhealthy ingredients?

SERVES 6 TO 8

---

2 pounds red beets, peeled, rinsed, and cut into ½-inch cubes

¼ cup olive oil, plus 2 tablespoons for roasting the beets

Salt and freshly ground black pepper

1 large shallot, minced

1 tablespoon whole-grain mustard

½ cup fresh orange juice

¼ cup fresh lemon juice

8 ounces carrots, peeled, rinsed, and finely grated (about 1 cup), packed

1 large crisp apple, cored and finely diced

½ cup toasted walnuts, roughly chopped

Leaves from 1 small bunch of fresh parsley, finely chopped

Leaves from 1 small bunch of fresh cilantro, finely chopped

Preheat the oven to 375°F and line a baking sheet with a double layer of aluminum foil.

In a mixing bowl, toss the beet chunks with 2 tablespoons of the olive oil and season generously with salt and pepper. Transfer the beets to the baking sheet, wrap the beets loosely in the foil, and roast them until tender, about 25 minutes. Set aside to cool.

To make the dressing, whisk together the ¼ cup olive oil, shallot, mustard, orange juice, and lemon juice. Season with salt and pepper to taste.

Toss the beets, carrots, apple, walnuts, parsley, and cilantro together in a large mixing bowl. Pour the dressing into the beet mixture and toss gently until well coated.

Roasted Beets with Anise, Cinnamon, and Orange Juice

This is an exotic but very simple riff on roasted beets. The licorice flavor of the anise complements the earthy flavor of the beets, and the cinnamon and orange juice both highlight the natural sweetness of the beets.

SERVES 4 TO 6

---

1 ½ pounds beets, peeled, rinsed, and cut into roughly 2-inch chunks

3 tablespoons olive oil

¼ teaspoon salt

½ teaspoon anise seeds

3 large cinnamon sticks, broken in half

⅓ cup good-quality orange juice

Preheat the oven to 375°F and line a roasting pan with a double layer of aluminum foil.

Toss all the ingredients together in the roasting pan and cover loosely with another piece of foil. Roast the beets, shaking a couple times along the way, until fork-tender, about 45 minutes.

in the raw

The easiest way to eat beets is in the raw. Get a cheap plastic Japanese mandoline at a kitchen store, wash and peel your beets, and thinly slice them on the mandoline. Arrange the slices on a plate, top with olive oil, salt, pepper, and a squeeze of lemon juice, and *voilà!* you have yourself a little beet snack.

Beet and Zucchini "Lasagne"

Beets and zucchini fill in for noodles in this "lasagne," which could easily become vegetarian by simply leaving out the ground meat. Though it's a whole lot tastier with it. SERVES 6

¼ cup olive oil

1 pound ground beef, preferably 95 percent lean

Salt and freshly ground black pepper

½ teaspoon hot red pepper flakes

1 teaspoon dried oregano

6 garlic cloves, minced or pressed

One 16-ounce can crushed tomatoes

1½ cups fresh ricotta cheese

⅛ teaspoon freshly grated nutmeg

2 pounds red beets, boiled, peeled (see page 55), and sliced ⅛ inch thick

3 medium zucchini, peeled lengthwise into ribbons down to the seeds

8 ounces mozzarella cheese, grated (about 2 cups)

Preheat the oven to 375°F.

Heat the oil in a large skillet over high heat. Add the ground beef, season very well with salt and pepper, and brown well, using a wooden spoon to break it up so that it forms small, even crumbles. Reduce the heat to medium-high and add the hot red pepper flakes, oregano, garlic, and tomatoes. Cook for 15 minutes; then remove from the heat and set aside to cool.

Combine the ricotta and nutmeg in a large mixing bowl and season with salt and pepper to taste.

Spread a spoonful of the beef sauce over the bottom of a glass baking dish roughly 7 × 11 inches. Layer on a quarter of the beets and zucchini, followed by a third of the ricotta mixture and a third of the remaining beef sauce. Repeat the layering, ending with a layer of beets and zucchini on top. Top this final layer with the mozzarella and bake for about 30 minutes, until bubbly and golden brown on top. Let cool slightly before cutting.

vitamins and food pairing

Cook up a beet lasagne and you'll get not only a hearty and healthy dinner but also a lesson in how to pair foods more effectively.

Beets are a good source of iron. But iron comes in two forms: heme iron, which is found in meats, poultry, and seafood, and nonheme iron, the kind in fruits, vegetables, and grains. The problem for people who limit their meat intake and rely on iron from other sources is that our bodies typically absorb only a small fraction of the nonheme iron found in plant-based foods. But pairing these foods with others that are rich in vitamin C enhances the body's ability to absorb iron.

Studies show that adding 25 milligrams of vitamin C to a meal can double the percentage of nonheme iron absorbed by the body and that 50 milligrams can more than triple it.

The lesson: Always try to combine nonheme sources of iron with foods that are high in vitamin C for maximum iron absorption. Think, for example, of a bowl of iron-enriched cereal (nonheme iron) mixed with strawberries (vitamin C) or a baked potato (nonheme iron) paired with a side of steamed broccoli (vitamin C).

Which is why the beets and tomatoes in this "lasagne" go hand in hand. One cup of tomato sauce alone is packed with about 26 milligrams of vitamin C—plenty of C to aid the iron content of the beets.

Fresh Beet Pappardelle with White Wine, Goat Cheese, and Thyme

Making fresh pasta is one of the joys of home cooking. Adding in beets is even more fun because of the colorful pasta you can create. The classic pairing of goat cheese and beets is played up in this recipe. No special equipment, except for a rolling pin, is required, but you could even use a wine bottle in a pinch! SERVES 4

For the Pasta:

8 ounces red beets, boiled, peeled (see page 55), and quartered

2 eggs

2 cups all-purpose flour, or more as needed

½ teaspoon fine salt

For the Sauce:

¼ cup olive oil

I large shallot, minced

I cup dry white wine

I teaspoon fresh thyme leaves, plus a couple teaspoons more for garnish

4 ounces soft goat cheese

Salt and freshly ground black pepper

Freshly grated Parmesan cheese to taste

Puree the beets and eggs in a blender or food processor until smooth. Whisk the flour and salt together in a large mixing bowl. Make a well in the flour and pour the beet puree into it. Mix the dry and wet ingredients together with a wooden spoon until you form a moist dough. If necessary, continue to add flour, ¼ cup at a time, until the dough is no longer sticky, but be careful not to add too much flour, as you could dry out the dough. Wrap the dough in plastic wrap and refrigerate overnight or for at least an hour.

Cut the ball of dough evenly into quarters and roll each one into a ball. Flour a metal or stone work surface very generously and on this surface roll out each ball with a rolling pin into as thin a sheet as possible without creating any breaks or holes. With a sharp knife, cut the sheets lengthwise into 1-inch-wide strips.

Bring a large pot of salted water to a boil. Cooking half of the strips of dough at a time, drop the strips into the boiling water, stirring gently from time to time, until they float to the top of the water, no more than 3 or 4 minutes. The pasta should appear cooked but still be a bit firm. Use a slotted spoon or a spider to remove the cooked pasta and transfer it to a bowl. Cook the remaining pasta and add it to the bowl.

To make the sauce, heat the oil in a small skillet over medium heat, add the shallot, and cook until fragrant and soft, just a couple minutes. Add the white wine and cook until reduced by half, about 5 minutes. Whisk in the thyme leaves and goat cheese until the mixture is smooth. Season with salt and pepper to taste. Pour the sauce over the pasta and toss. Garnish with Parmesan and some more fresh thyme.

Beet and Caramelized Onion Potato Mash

This is a tasty take on potato mash with a healthy kick from all the beets in the mix. It's a versatile side dish that can go with just about anything from fish to beef to chicken. The caramelized onions make the mash deliciously sweet and rich. SERVES 6

2½ pounds starchy potatoes, such as russet or Yukon Gold, peeled and quartered

Salt and freshly ground black pepper

¼ cup olive oil

I large yellow onion, halved lengthwise and thinly sliced crosswise

I pound red beets, boiled, peeled (see page 55), and quartered

I small bunch of fresh chives, finely chopped

Put the potatoes in a large pot of heavily salted cold water. Bring the water to a boil and simmer the potatoes until fork-tender, about 25 minutes.

In a large skillet, heat the oil over medium heat. Add the sliced onion and cook, stirring often, until caramelized, 12 to 15 minutes. Remove from the heat.

Strain the water from the pot and add the beets and caramelized onion to the potatoes. Mash well. Season to taste with the salt and pepper and finish by sprinkling in the chives.

Yellow Beet and Apricot Curry

A pretty yellow riff on curry in which the sweetness of the apricots and the beets truly shines through. I go pretty light on the curry powder, so I don't completely overwhelm the more subtle flavors of the beets, but if you want a spicier dish, feel free to add a few more teaspoons. You can serve this curry over brown rice, but for an extra protein kick substitute quinoa. SERVES 6

---

3 tablespoons olive oil

I large onion, coarsely grated

3 garlic cloves, minced

2 tablespoons grated fresh ginger

I small red bell pepper, finely chopped

2 tablespoons tomato paste

I tablespoon plus I teaspoon yellow curry powder

½ cup dried apricots, roughly chopped

1½ cups chicken or vegetable stock

½ cup coconut milk

I pound yellow beets, boiled, peeled (see page 55), and cut into eighths

Salt and freshly ground black pepper

I small bunch of scallions, thinly sliced

I small bunch of cilantro, roughly chopped

Heat the olive oil in a large skillet over medium heat. Add the onion, garlic, ginger, and red pepper, cover, and cook, stirring frequently, about 7 minutes. Add the tomato paste, curry powder, and apricots and cook for 5 minutes longer. Add the stock and coconut milk, bring to a simmer, and cook for about 10 minutes. Add the beets and cook for 5 minutes longer. Season with salt and pepper to taste and finish by topping with the scallions and cilantro.

Beef and Beet Stew

This is my take on borscht, the classic Eastern European beet soup. It is a delicious, hearty soup that melds the richness of the beef with the sweetness of the beets. The longer you cook the broth, the more delicious your stew will be. SERVES 6 TO 8

2 pounds boneless beef round, cut into roughly 1-inch pieces

2 large carrots, roughly chopped

3 celery stalks, roughly chopped

3 medium onions, quartered

4 ounces tomato paste

Kosher salt

1 tablespoon black peppercorns

3 bay leaves

5 fresh thyme sprigs

1 pound red beets, peeled and grated

1 pound white cabbage, shredded

1 pound russet potatoes, peeled and finely diced

¼ cup red wine vinegar, plus more to finish

4 large garlic cloves, finely chopped

1 small bunch of fresh dill, stems removed and roughly chopped

Freshly ground black pepper

Combine the beef, carrots, celery, onions, tomato paste, 2 tablespoons salt, the peppercorns, bay leaves, and thyme in a large stockpot and add water to cover by 4 or 5 inches. Bring to a simmer. After about 30 minutes, skim off any foam from the top, reduce the heat to the lowest setting, and cook, partially covered, for about 4 hours.

Strain the broth through a fine-mesh sieve into another large pot, return the beef to the broth, and discard the vegetables. Add the beets, cabbage, potatoes, vinegar, chopped garlic, and a handful of dill. Cook for 30 minutes longer, or until the potatoes are fork-tender. Finish by adding the remaining dill and season to taste with salt, ground pepper, and vinegar.

got beef?

We know what you're thinking: What on earth is red meat doing in a book of healthy recipes?

If it seems as out of place as a soyburger in a steakhouse, trust us—it's not. The news about red meat these days may seem entirely frightening—after all, it's been linked to heart disease, high cholesterol, and colorectal cancer—but research shows that lean beef can have a place in a healthy diet. In fact it may even improve health. It provides protein, selenium, zinc, iron, phosphorus, and B vitamins, all without the saturated fat that weighs down other cuts. And, if it's organic, it'll spare you the pesticides, hormones, and antibiotics found in nonorganic meat.

Strip away the fat, and you're left with a lean source of nutrients, including conjugated linoleic acid, or CLA, a natural fatty acid that's been shown to have beneficial properties. No surprise then that studies of large populations of heavy meat eaters show that consuming mostly fatty cuts of red meat significantly increases the risk of colorectal cancer, while consuming mostly lean beef has the reverse effect, sharply decreasing your risk.

And studies of heart disease have had similarly encouraging results. People with high cholesterol who were started on lean beef, lean fish, or poultry diets reduced their levels of LDL, or bad, cholesterol by about 10 percent and increased their levels of the good, HDL cholesterol. A lean-fish diet was still far better at raising HDL cholesterol levels than a lean-beef diet, but the underlying point is that for those with a ravenous carnivore in them, lean beef can reward more than just the taste buds.

Mix it up with the beets and tomatoes in the stew and you might find even more benefits. The iron in the beef, of the heme iron variety, increases the absorption of the nonheme iron in the beets, which is typically not easily absorbed. Same goes for the vitamin C in the tomatoes, a potent iron enhancer.

Some readily available cuts of lean beef include cuts from the round, shoulder, and rump, as well as flank steak.

Chocolate Beet Mini-Cakes

These cakes are light, moist, and delicious. Using high-quality Dutch-process cocoa will give you a dark, rich, and chocolaty cupcake. Though you won't be able to tell that beets are even in the mix, a mere ½ pound in each batch makes the cupcakes extra moist. And if you're trying to sneak beets into every aspect of your family's diet without causing a stir, this is definitely the way to go! MAKES 18 MINI-CAKES

1 cup whole wheat flour

⅔ cup Dutch-process cocoa powder

1½ teaspoons baking powder

½ teaspoon baking soda

⅛ teaspoon fine salt

3 large eggs

1¼ cups sugar

1 cup canola oil

½ pound red beets, boiled, peeled (see page 55), and finely grated

½ cup yogurt

Preheat the oven to 325°F and line an 18-muffin tin with foil cups.

Whisk the flour, cocoa, baking powder, baking soda, and salt together in one bowl and the remaining ingredients in another. Gradually mix the dry ingredients into the egg mixture. Fill each muffin cup half full with the mixture.

Bake for 20 minutes, or until a toothpick inserted into the center of a mini-cake comes out clean and the mini-cakes start to pull away from the sides of the tin. Cool before serving.

Muffins will keep for 2 days in an airtight container at room temperature.

beets, canola oil, whole wheat flour?

Not the sort of ingredients that typically make for unforgettable desserts, sinfully enjoyed. But in our world, it's possible to transform a set of healthful ingredients into a plate of hearty indulgence.

For starters, forget about butter, with its artery-impeding fats. Here we're swapping in canola oil: low in saturated fat, high in the good monounsaturated kind, and containing some omega-3s for good measure. Then we push aside the out-of-date refined flour; nutritious whole wheat flour brings this cake up to date. On top of that, we cut back on the sugar. The natural sweetness of beets gives us a little boost.

But what about the chocolate? you ask. Despite what's often assumed, chocolate is not exactly a health disaster—particularly dark chocolate, which is free of the butterfat that goes into milk chocolate. Besides brimming with antioxidants—the same ones found in red wine and tea—chocolate contains compounds that are known to raise the spirits. One of these compounds, tryptophan, is a precursor to serotonin, which creates feelings of pleasure and plays a role in sexual arousal. Another, theobromine, is a stimulant that elevates mood, and a third, phenylethylamine, is released in the brain when people fall in love.

According to studies, it's unclear whether these three chemicals are plentiful enough to produce measurable effects on mood. But the brain is our largest sexual organ, and psychologists argue that anything that stirs feelings of warmth, satisfaction, and pleasure can have strong aphrodisiac effects on the mind—including comfort food. So why not break these out on Valentine's Day or for a special date night?

Unlike other comfort foods, these cupcakes should be eaten with lots of love and little guilt.

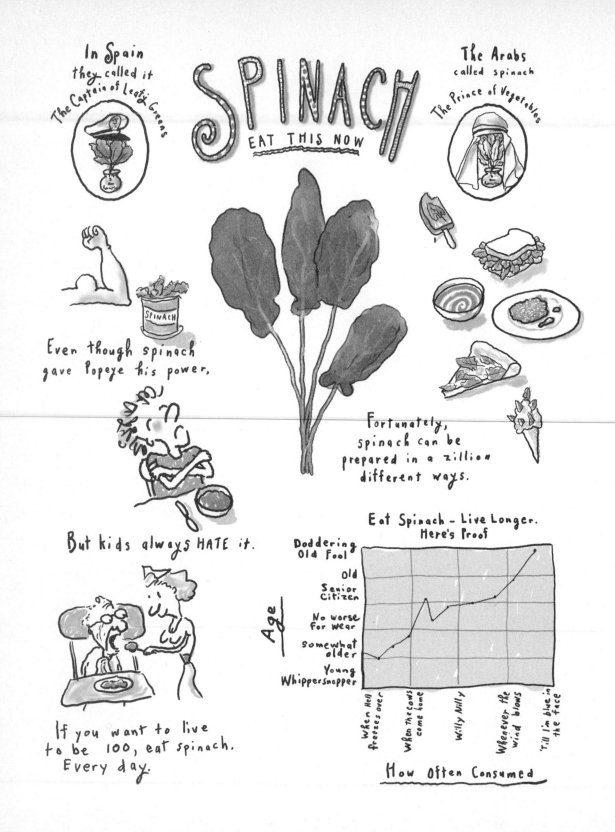

4

SPINACH

A mantra in the health world is that no single food can ensure better health. It takes a balanced diet, the thinking goes, and a team of wholesome foods to shield you from disease and the wear and tear of aging. But every winning team has its star player. And on an all-star lineup of healthy foods, spinach would easily be the MVP. This is a food that is not only nutritionally outstanding but one so powerful it has been celebrated across cultures for thousands of years.

The vegetable has its roots in ancient Persia, the cradle of civilization, and has been loved nearly everywhere it has turned up since. The Spanish called spinach "the captain of leafy greens." The Arabs called it "the prince of vegetables." And the king of Nepal in the seventh century adored spinach so much that he single-handedly introduced it to China when he sent it to the country as a gesture of goodwill. In Renaissance France, soldiers were served wine fortified with spinach juice to help them recover from severe wounds.

And yet, in America, spinach has long been saddled by a terrible rep. "One man's poison ivy is another man's spinach," George Ade, the turn-of-the-century humorist, once quipped. Or as Delia Ephron, the noted writer, once observed, the way to eat spinach is to "divide into little piles. Rearrange again into new piles. After five or six maneuvers, sit back and say you are full."

But the reality is that you just can't find another food that's packed with more nutrition, flavor, and potential as an ingredient. If spinach came with a slogan, it would be three words: eat this now!

Forget for a moment everything you ever learned about spinach, right down to the cartoonish depictions you saw as a child. We all grew up watching cartoons of Popeye guzzling spinach by the can so he could sprout enormous biceps and rescue his beloved "goyl." That perception was rooted in the idea that spinach is loaded with muscle-building iron, which is rather misleading. Spinach contains plenty of iron, but it's not the kind that is easily absorbed, unless it happens to be paired with other foods that contain vitamin C.

The real beauty of spinach is not what it builds but what it destroys. Spinach is overflowing with a lineup of compounds that have funny names—names you wouldn't want to pronounce, like neoxanthin and kaempferol—and that all have one very serious thing in common: they are kryptonite to cancer cells.

It's a phenomenon that has been demonstrated over and over. As the amount of spinach in a person's diet goes up, the risk of cancer goes down.

The evidence of this is sitting on my desk at home in the form of a massive binder stuffed with papers. Inside are countless studies from countries around the world, each attesting to the fact that a diet heavy in spinach can extinguish the risk of an impressive array of cancers: prostate, ovarian, colorectal, breast, bladder, stomach, and esophageal, to name just a few.

Flip through this huge body of evidence and you'll find, for example, a 2007 study by the National Cancer Institute. Nearly half a million people were involved, about as large a group of subjects as you're ever going to find. The scientists scrutinized every detail of the participants' diets, taking inventory of everything they ate and examining every aspect of their daily behaviors, from exercise to alcohol intake and cigarette smoking. In this case, after controlling for all of these variables and more, they chose to look specifically at the rates of esophageal cancer, a virulent form of cancer that has a notoriously low survival rate. The end result was clear: "A significant inverse association between esophageal adenocarcinoma and spinach intake was observed."

That's characteristically dry scientific language for: "Eat more spinach, and keep the Big C at bay."

That is the sort of news that should make any American perk up and listen. In the United States, cancer has long been a leading killer, second only to heart disease. One out of three Americans alive today will get a cancer diagnosis, and every year more than a million new cases are confirmed. We all know someone who has fought a battle with this devastating disease.

No one is saying that spinach—or any food for that matter—is a silver bullet. But with a body of evidence so compelling, it would be foolish not to make spinach a regular part of your diet. And if you live in America, chances are you could use some more vegetables on your plate. According to the Centers for Disease Control and Prevention, fewer than three out of ten Americans eat at least three vegetables a day, the minimum recommended by the USDA. Statistics like that might help explain why at least half of the ten leading causes of death in the United States are conditions that have some link to diet: heart disease, cancer, stroke, Alzheimer's, and diabetes.

For the seven out of ten Americans who need to step up their vegetable intake, spinach is a clever choice. It contains so many antioxidants that in some ways it's the equivalent of two or three servings of vegetables in one.

How do we know this? Because fifteen years ago, scientists at the National Institutes of Health came up with a nifty way of measuring a food's antioxidant power. Called the *oxygen radical absorbance capacity*, this measurement indicates a food's ability to rid the body of free radicals, the harmful molecular fragments that have been linked to aging and chronic disease. As with a popularity poll, the higher a food's ORAC value, the better.

According to the USDA, a serving of celery has an ORAC value of 497. That's not bad. Carrots come in at 666 units per serving. That's better still. But step aside and make room for spinach. A single serving soars off the charts, with an ORAC value of 1,515.

And that comes on top of everything else that Mother Nature has crammed into those crisp green leaves: calcium, potassium, vitamin K, vitamin A, folate, omega-3s, and a slew of other nutrients.

All of which begs the question: is spinach on *your* dinner plate?

If you still aren't convinced, it may be instructive to look at what's on the plates in the parts of the world where good health and long life are part of the culture. In the countries that have the world's highest concentrations of centenarians, it may be no surprise that spinach has long been on the daily menu.

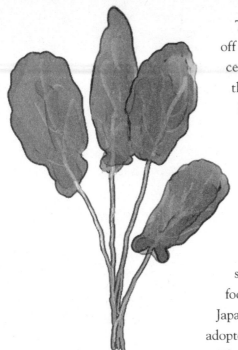

Take a spin through the islands of Okinawa just off the coast of northern Japan. The percentage of centenarians here is several times greater than in the rest of Japan, which already has the longest life expectancy of any nation in the world. The traditional breakfast in Okinawa is a bowl of miso with spinach and egg. Okinawans love their spinach, as well as other leafy green vegetables, which they eat multiple times a day. As a result they have long experienced some of the lowest rates of heart disease and cancer of any region in the world (this has started to change only in recent years, as fast-food outlets like McDonald's have spread across Japan and younger Okinawans have increasingly adopted a Western diet).

Thousands of miles away in the Mediterranean Sea sits another longevity hot spot: Sardinia, a sun-drenched island off the coast of Italy. One out of every 200 people living in this island's eastern province of Ogliastra celebrates a hundredth birthday, about fifty times the rate in the United States. Take a seat at a dinner table in this sunny oasis and you'll almost certainly find a centuries-old specialty and dietary staple called *culingiones*—round ravioli stuffed with spinach and fresh ricotta. If the main course on this particular evening includes a cut of lean meat, chances are it'll be paired with sautéed spinach and potatoes, a favorite side dish.

After a quick stop in Sardinia, take a short flight over to Greece, the country that gave us the original heart-healthy Mediterranean diet. You won't find a dinner table here that doesn't have some version of spinach and feta cheese, spinach croquettes, or one of my all-time favorites, spinach pie (*spanakopita*, as we Americans know it).

So how can you make your plate look more like a centenarian's? Dumping a small pile of spinach beside every meal is one quick way, but that alone wouldn't do much to please the palate, and a habit that boring would be hard to sustain. The key, as Dave points out, is to prepare spinach in a way that makes the taste buds flutter:

Making spinach taste good is really much simpler than people think. The bad rep that spinach has had in this country for so long is primarily based around the idea that spinach tastes nasty. Children are expected to look at the stuff and make all kinds of disturbing faces. But why? In reality, spinach is one of the most versatile, sweet, and mild greens out there. I can't think of another leafy green that can be enjoyed in so many states—raw, steamed, sautéed, or as an element in a limitless array of dishes—and together with such a variety of seasoning and preparations.

Maybe it's just that people who have an aversion to spinach have been cooking it incorrectly all this time. Or should I say overcooking it?

See, when you cook spinach too long, it actually can get a little unpleasant. Overcooked spinach can get slimy. It loses its healthy bright green color, and it can even take on a metallic or bitter taste. But there is a simple solution to this problem, leaving you with sweet, delicious spinach every time—just cook it quickly! No matter how you decide to cook spinach, it doesn't need more than a couple minutes to reach perfect doneness. Of course there are exceptions to this rule: with some variation, creamy long-cooked spinach dishes are enjoyed all over the world, from deep in the American South to dinner tables in India. But for the most part, you'll get the best flavor out of spinach if you cook it just until it is tender and wilted while still hanging on to its vibrant green color.

Chefs know this, of course, and the way most chefs achieve perfectly cooked spinach is by blanching it, which involves submerging it briefly in boiling water and then transferring it immediately to a bath of ice water to stop the spinach from cooking any further. But this can be a bit of a pain to do in the home kitchen and, as I learned from Anahad, when you boil spinach some of those incredibly beneficial nutrients and antioxidants leach into the cooking water and wind up down the kitchen drain rather than in your body, which sounds to me like throwing the baby out with the bathwater. So I played around with steaming spinach (which works well), but microwaving spinach that has been rinsed and left a bit wet works wonders. I've written a quick description of the process for you to try your hand at it.

In coming up with recipes for this chapter I wanted to highlight just how versatile spinach truly is, so you'll find spinach prepared in all kinds of ways, from flash-sautéed to whizzed in a blender. If you work your way through these recipes, I think you'll find that spinach is not only a health wonder but a culinary one too.

Mixed Bean, Barley, and Spinach Soup

I've kept this hearty soup simple to allow the honest, earthy flavors of all the vegetables to come through. SERVES 8

½ cup dried kidney beans

½ cup dried pinto beans

½ cup dried navy beans

1 large onion, finely chopped

2 medium carrots, finely chopped

2 large celery stalks, finely chopped

1 quart chicken or vegetable stock

3 bay leaves

1 teaspoon dried oregano

½ cup green split peas

½ cup barley

1 pound fresh spinach, tough stems removed, roughly torn

2 teaspoons Tabasco sauce

Salt and freshly ground black pepper

Combine the beans, vegetables, stock, 1 quart water, the bay leaves, and the dried oregano in a large pot. Bring to a simmer over high heat; then reduce the heat to low, cover, and cook, stirring occasionally, until the beans are tender, about 1 hour.

Add the split peas and barley and cook until the peas and barley are soft, another 30 minutes. Add the spinach leaves, pushing them down into the soup to wilt, cover the pot, and cook for 15 minutes longer. Stir in the Tabasco sauce and season with salt and pepper to taste.

Store in an air-tight container in the refrigerator up to a week or in the freezer for up to a month.

retaining spinach goodness through proper cooking and storage

It's hard to find a vegetable with more nutrients than spinach. But cook or store it the wrong way and it loses much of its power.

Rule number one: Never boil your spinach. Because boiling strips away many water-soluble vitamins—and dark, leafy greens are loaded with them—throwing your spinach in a pot of hot water is a quick way to wash away those nutrients. In studies at Cornell University, scientists found that boiling spinach causes it to lose nearly 80 percent of its folate. But steaming, stir-frying, and microwaving have almost no impact.

In fact, stir-frying may be more beneficial than eating your spinach raw: The added oil helps your body absorb antioxidants like beta-carotene.

Whenever possible, try not to keep your spinach sitting around in the refrigerator too long. While some fruits and vegetables are fine when kept in the cooler, spinach starts losing its vitamins and minerals almost as soon as it's pulled from the ground. And after a week of refrigeration, it loses almost 50 percent of its folate and more than half of its amount of antioxidants like lutein.

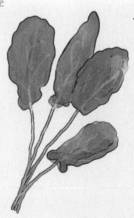

If you can't avoid storage time, simply opt for the frozen variety, which retains more of its nutrients.

Sautéed Sesame Spinach

Asian cuisines know that spinach can handle their most potent seasonings, like soy sauce and dark sesame oil. I took a page from these cooks to toss together this dish and added a little Italian twist of the wrist with the balsamic vinegar, which gives the spinach a sweet and tangy touch.

SERVES 4 TO 6

2 tablespoons dark sesame oil

2 tablespoons canola oil

2 large bunches of fresh spinach, stem ends trimmed

2 tablespoons soy sauce

1 tablespoon Asian fish sauce

3 garlic cloves, thinly sliced

2 tablespoons balsamic vinegar

2 tablespoons sesame seeds

Heat the oils in a large skillet over high heat until they shimmer. Rinse the spinach in cold water, quickly shake off the excess water, and then use tongs to work the leaves through the hot oil. Once the spinach has wilted down, add the soy sauce, fish sauce, garlic, and vinegar and cook for 4 to 5 minutes longer, stirring frequently.

To serve, transfer the sautéed spinach to a serving bowl and sprinkle the sesame seeds over the top.

Sweet Curried Spinach
and Chickpeas

I love the way Indian cuisine often combines spinach with chickpeas. Here's a simple riff on that idea. Adding just a touch of sweetness to the dish makes this combination nearly addictive, which isn't something you hear too often about either spinach or chickpeas! SERVES 4 TO 6

3 tablespoons canola oil

1 large onion, finely chopped

1 tablespoon curry powder

2 tablespoons honey

1 cup chicken or vegetable stock, preferably homemade

Two 15-ounce cans chickpeas, drained

20 ounces frozen spinach, thawed

Salt

Heat the oil in a large skillet over medium heat. Add the onion and cook, stirring often, until softened and nearly translucent, about 7 minutes. Stir in the curry powder and honey and cook together for a couple minutes. Add the stock, chickpeas, and spinach. Bring the mixture to a simmer and cook for 15 minutes longer. Season with salt to taste.

microwave blanching

One of the most common ways of preparing spinach for use is to blanch it, which means briefly dropping fresh spinach into a pot of boiling water, just long enough for it to wilt and turn bright green. But seeing that so much of spinach's nutrient goodness is lost through this method, we turn to other cooking methods: steaming and microwaving.

Steaming a bunch of spinach is fairly easy and works like a charm, but microwaving spinach works just as well and is even faster and easier.

Here's all you have to do:

Rinse the spinach to be blanched and shake off as much of the excess water as possible. It shouldn't be completely dry, though, because this remaining moisture will essentially steam the spinach in the microwave.

Place the rinsed spinach in a microwave-safe bowl or container large enough to comfortably hold the amount of spinach at hand. Cover with a tight-fitting lid or a large plate.

Zap for 2 to 3 minutes on high power (depending on the quantity of spinach), stirring once in the middle of the cooking time.

When the spinach has wilted into one soft, wet, bright green lump, you know you're ready to go!

Spinach Quiche

Most quiches call for crusts filled with processed flours and loads of butter. But this delicious and hearty whole wheat crust doesn't leave you missing the traditional version at all. And you won't have to mess around with pie weights or bags of dried beans as you often have to with the butter and white flour versions. MAKES ONE 9-INCH QUICHE, SERVING 6 TO 8

For the Crust:

2 cups whole wheat flour

½ teaspoon salt

¼ cup olive oil

½ cup ice water

For the Filling:

¼ cup canola oil

1 large onion, finely chopped

4 ounces speck, finely chopped (optional)

10 ounces frozen spinach, thawed

Salt and freshly ground black pepper

8 large eggs

1 ounce Parmesan or pecorino cheese, grated (about ¼ cup), plus more for garnish

⅛ teaspoon freshly grated nutmeg

Preheat the oven to 350°F.

To make the crust, stir the flour, salt, and olive oil together in a large mixing bowl. Gradually mix in the ice water, until the mixture starts to pull together to form a loose ball. Trickle in a little more ice water if necessary. Use your hands to pat the mixture into a firm ball, wrap in plastic wrap, and chill in the refrigerator for at least 30 minutes.

To make the filling, heat the canola oil in a large skillet over medium-high heat. Add the onion and cook, partially covered, stirring often, until softened and translucent, about 7 minutes. Add the speck and spinach and cook for 5 minutes longer. Season with salt and pepper to taste. Set aside to cool.

Break the eggs into a large mixing bowl and beat well. Stir in the cheese, nutmeg, ½ teaspoon salt, and ½ teaspoon pepper. Stir in the cooled spinach mixture.

Unwrap the chilled ball of dough and place on a clean, well-floured work surface. Use a rolling pin to roll out the dough into a disk about ¼ inch thick and 9 or 10 inches in diameter. Press the dough into a 9-inch Pyrex pie plate. Use a small fork to make a bunch of shallow dents in the bottom of the crust.

Bake the crust for 15 minutes; then remove it from the oven, pour in the egg and spinach mixture, and bake for about 35 minutes longer, until the center is firm to the touch and the top has browned lightly. Allow to cool for at least 10 minutes before serving so the quiche holds together when sliced. Before serving, garnish with more freshly grated cheese if you like.

Spinach and Lamb Farfalle

You might find a recipe like this in a southern Italian farmhouse. If you don't eat lamb, you can substitute any other kind of ground meat. SERVES 4

¼ cup olive oil, plus more for drizzling

I pound ground lamb

Salt and freshly ground black pepper

I small onion, finely chopped

8 ounces spinach farfalle

5 garlic cloves, minced

10 ounces frozen chopped spinach, thawed

Juice of I lemon

4 ounces reduced-fat goat cheese, crumbled, plus more for garnish

I bunch of fresh mint, stems removed and leaves finely chopped, plus more for garnish

12 prunes, finely chopped

2 tablespoons pine nuts

I tablespoon honey

Bring a large pot of water to a boil for the pasta. Heat the oil in a large skillet over medium-high heat. Add the lamb, season generously with salt and pepper, and cook, breaking up the meat with a wooden spoon until brown and crumbled, about 5 minutes. Add the chopped onion and cook for 5 minutes longer, stirring often. Add the pasta to the boiling water with some salt and cook al dente. Drain the pasta, reserving a little pasta water. In the skillet, add the garlic, spinach, and lemon juice to the sauce and cook for another 5 minutes. Add the remaining ingredients and cook until the cheese has melted, about 3 minutes. Toss with the drained pasta.

If the mixture looks dry, add a few tablespoons of the reserved pasta water. Garnish with more of the mint and the crumbled goat cheese, and drizzle with the olive oil.

spinach and mental health

Spinach may not give you bigger muscles. But would you settle for a stronger brain?

Compounds in spinach have been shown in studies to have a remarkably protective effect on the brain, keeping at bay the normal cognitive and motor declines that come with aging.

Take it from the National Institute of Aging and Rush University Medical Center. In 2006 they published a study of nearly four thousand elderly adults, looking closely at how their diets affected their mental faculties as they aged.

Ultimately they found that over time people who ate just three servings of vegetables a day saw a 40 percent slower decline in mental performance than people who ate less than one serving. But the greatest protection was seen in people who ate spinach and other dark green leafy vegetables. Compared with their spinach-abstaining counterparts, they were able to shed about five years from their noggins.

The antioxidants that do the job are best absorbed in the presence of fat, which is why you'll find plenty of olive oil in (and drizzled on top of) our combination of spinach and lamb over spinach farfalle. Don't be shy with the olive oil. The more the better. And we've added plenty of heart-healthy fats—like canola oil—to our other spinach recipes for the same reason.

Spinach Linguine with Spinach Arugula and Walnut Pesto

Pestos are generally packed with all kinds of ingredients that are good for you. Here I'm taking it up a level by adding plenty of spinach, lots of heart-healthy walnuts, and a good bunch of spicy arugula, which comes through nicely in the finished dish. SERVES 6

---

3 ounces baby arugula

5 ounces fresh spinach, microwave-blanched (see page 84)

½ cup olive oil, plus more for drizzling

Juice of 1 lemon

½ cup finely grated Parmesan cheese, plus more for garnish

½ cup walnut halves

2 garlic cloves, peeled

Salt and freshly ground pepper

1 pound spinach linguine

Bring a large pot of water to a boil for the pasta. Meanwhile, combine 2 ounces of the arugula with the blanched spinach, ½ cup olive oil, lemon juice, ½ cup Parmesan, walnuts, garlic, 1 teaspoon salt, and a generous amount of pepper in a blender and blend until smooth. Add a little water to the mixture if blending is troublesome.

Add a little salt to the boiling water and cook the linguine al dente. Drain and toss with the pesto.

To serve, divide the pasta among 6 bowls, top each with a small handful of the remaining arugula, and use a peeler to shave more Parmesan over the top of each portion. Finish with a drizzle of the olive oil.

getting kids to eat spinach

Spinach may be a hall-of-fame power food, but any parent of a picky child knows it can be notoriously difficult to get children to eat it.

Forget trying to sneak it into their food. Here's a more effective way, endorsed by scientific research: just tell them they loved eating it as younger children.

Deceptively simple, but it works.

Psychologists at the University of California, Irvine, have conducted studies in which they were able to get college students to eat vegetables they previously hated—and to balk at foods they previously loved—simply by implanting false memories. In one study in 2008, they recruited dozens of college students and had them fill out detailed questionnaires about their food histories, telling them they were part of a study on food preferences and personality. Then they selected the subjects who rated asparagus the most negatively and said they had always avoided it.

A week later, these students were told that a sophisticated computer-generated analysis of their childhood experiences determined, among other things, that they had liked to eat cooked asparagus as children. Ultimately, this information made most of the asparagus-hating students significantly more willing to buy and eat it in the future. Swapping spinach for asparagus should have the same effect.

In other studies, the same psychologists used similar tricks to convince young adults that various foods they enjoyed, from pickles to hard-boiled eggs and strawberry ice cream, had made them sick as children. The result? They were less likely to eat these foods in the future.

The reason this works is that memories tend to be constructed, not played back in the style of a videotape, which means they can easily be altered by the power of suggestion. If it means telling a small white lie to get your kids to eat healthier, isn't it worth it?

Grilled Fish with Tangy Spinach, Cilantro, and Caper Puree

Any meaty fish, such as mahimahi or salmon, pairs well with this puree. I used mako shark, which is quite readily available, but you can play around with another fish you like so long as it is hearty enough to hold up on the grill. SERVES 6

For the Fish:

2 pounds meaty fish, cut into 6 large fillets

Salt and freshly ground black pepper

¼ cup canola oil

For the Sauce:

5 ounces baby spinach, microwave-blanched (see page 84)

1 bunch of cilantro, tough stems removed

2 tablespoons drained capers, plus more for garnish

1 garlic clove

¼ cup olive oil

¼ cup red wine vinegar or fresh lemon juice

½ teaspoon salt

Lemon wedges for serving

Preheat your grill or grill pan to high heat (you shouldn't be able to comfortably hold your hand a couple inches from the grill for more than 6 or 7 seconds).

Season the fish fillets generously with salt and pepper. Rub all over with the oil. Grill until the fish is white and cooked through, a few minutes per side. Set aside to rest briefly.

Combine all the ingredients for the sauce in a blender and blend until smooth.

Place the fillets on a large serving platter. Drizzle with the sauce, sprinkle with a handful of drained capers, and serve with the lemon wedges.

Chicken Scaloppine with Sweet and Sour Spinach

One of my favorite spinach pairings is the sweet and sour combination. A less substantial green would have trouble standing up to so much flavor, but, oh no, not spinach. SERVES 4

For the Chicken:

4 boneless, skinless chicken breasts (about 8 ounces each)

Salt and freshly ground black pepper

¼ cup all-purpose flour

¼ cup canola oil

For the Spinach:

⅓ cup balsamic vinegar

¼ cup red or golden raisins

I cup chicken stock

3 garlic cloves, finely chopped

One 15-ounce can cannellini beans, rinsed and drained

10 ounces fresh spinach, microwave-blanched (see page 84) and drained

½ cup walnut halves, toasted and roughly chopped

Place each chicken breast between 2 large sheets of plastic wrap. Use a meat mallet or heavy-bottomed pan to pound them to about a ½-inch thickness. Season generously with salt and pepper. Put the flour into a bowl and dredge each breast well to coat evenly.

Heat the oil in a large skillet over high heat. Fry the breasts, in batches if necessary, until crispy, browned, and cooked through, about 4 minutes per side. Set aside to rest.

Remove the cooled chicken from the pan and add the vinegar, raisins, stock, garlic, and beans. Bring to a simmer and cook until thickened, about 7 minutes. Add the spinach and cook just a couple minutes longer. Remove from the heat and stir in the walnuts. Serve each chicken breast with a side of the spinach.

Baby Spinach–Stuffed Matambre

I was first introduced to *matambre* not on a recent trip to Argentina but rather right here in New York City through my friends at the *Saveur* magazine test kitchen. I upped the amount of spinach traditionally used, so it is even better for you, but it still has the fantastic flavor I fell in love with. SERVES 6

4 small carrots, quartered lengthwise

Salt and freshly ground black pepper

I large flank steak (about 2 pounds)

10 ounces fresh spinach, microwave-blanched (see page 84)

I medium onion, halved lengthwise and thinly sliced crosswise

¼ cup canola oil

I quart chicken or beef stock

I bottle dry red wine

6 garlic cloves, smashed

½ teaspoon dried marjoram

½ teaspoon dried thyme

I large bay leaf

Put the sliced carrots in a large saucepan and cover with water by no more than an inch. Season generously with salt and bring to a simmer over medium-high heat. Cook the carrots until tender, about 15 minutes; drain and set aside to cool.

Put the flank steak between 2 large sheets of plastic wrap and use a meat mallet or heavy-bottomed pan to pound the meat to about a ¼-inch thickness. Remove the meat from the plastic wrap and season generously on both sides with salt and pepper.

Distribute the carrots, spinach, and onion on the flank steak, laying the carrots lengthwise down the length of the steak and leaving an inch of space free around the edge of the meat so that the filling doesn't spill out when it is rolled up.

Have a couple feet of butcher's twine ready. Use the long side to tightly roll the steak up. Make a series of tight knots around the roll to make a neat package.

Heat the canola oil in a large, heavy-bottomed Dutch oven over high heat. Brown the steak well on all sides. Pour off any excess oil; then add the stock, wine, garlic, and herbs. Bring to a simmer, reduce the heat to medium-low, and cook until the steak is very tender, about 3 hours.

To serve, allow the steak to cool on a cutting board for about 10 minutes. Use kitchen scissors to cut the twine and slice the steak crosswise into 6 portions. Serve each portion with a ladle of the cooking liquid poured over the top.

Mediterranean Baked Eggs

When was the last time you had eggs for dinner? Well, if it's been a while, wait no longer. This dish is savory, substantial, and presentable enough that you could easily serve it at a casual dinner party when a light meal or an interesting appetizer is in order. SERVES 6

¼ cup canola oil

8 ounces baby bella mushrooms, thinly sliced

1 large red onion, halved lengthwise and thinly sliced lengthwise

10 sun-dried tomatoes

10 ounces fresh spinach, microwave-blanched (see page 84)

Salt and freshly ground black pepper

6 eggs

½ cup finely grated Parmesan cheese

Preheat the oven to 350°F.

Heat the oil in a large skillet over high heat. Add the mushrooms and fry, stirring continuously, until the mushrooms have wilted and start to brown lightly, about 7 to 10 minutes. Reduce the heat to medium and add the onion and sun-dried tomatoes. Cook, partially covered, stirring often, until the onion is very soft and starting to take on some color, about 10 minutes longer. Stir in the blanched spinach and season with salt and pepper to taste.

Remove from the heat and use a rubber spatula or wooden spoon to distribute the mixture evenly around the pan while still leaving plenty of crags and nooks for the eggs to settle into. Crack the eggs, one by one, into a small bowl to check for shell fragments, then place directly on top of the spinach mixture, distributing the eggs evenly around the pan. Top the eggs with the cheese and move the skillet from the stovetop to the oven. Bake for 10 to 15 minutes, until the cheese has melted and the egg whites have set but the yolks are still runny. Serve immediately.

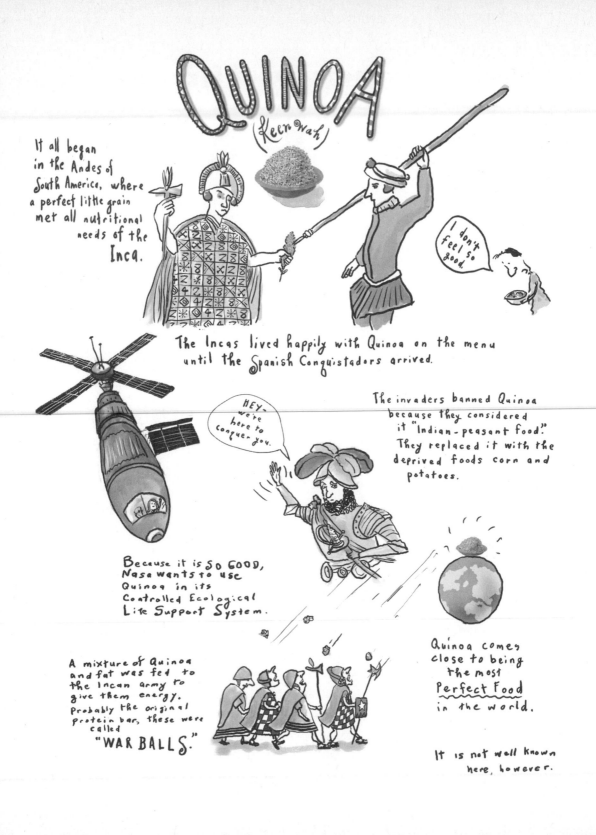

5

QUINOA

Across this massive planet of ours, in countries on every continent except Antarctica, thousands of varieties of grains sprout from millions of acres of farmland.

But what if you needed to survive on one, and only one, of these grains for the rest of your life? Which one would you choose to give your body nearly everything it needs to function? Would it be possible to find a grain so full of protein and fiber and minerals and healthy fats that you could make it a routine part of your diet and virtually forgo all other food?

It is a daunting thought.

"It must be brown rice!" you say—the veritable staple of every health-conscious American's diet that no health food store would be complete without. And indeed, brown rice is a supreme source of fiber, not to mention a slew of important minerals. But when it comes to protein, forget it. You'd be hard-pressed to find many amino acids stored in those crunchy little grains, and we all know that no one can get by without enough protein.

"OK!" you say then. "Barley must be the answer!" High in protein and a great source of fiber, it is an excellent food by any standards. But once again, it turns out that barley would leave you lacking magnesium and several other critical nutrients.

On to the next candidate. Oats are so versatile they're used in everything from breakfast cereals to porridge and even beer. You may remember the nationwide oat bran craze of the 1980s, fueled by the news that a diet high in oats could lower cholesterol. That may be true, but keep in mind that oats have the second-highest fat content of any cereal behind maize. When it comes to grains, there's much room for improvement.

As you see, this can be a maddening task so mystifying it would take a team of rocket scientists to figure it out. But as it happens, that's already been done.

In the 1990s, scientists at NASA set out to find the consummate grain, one that was so complete they could send it with astronauts on long-duration space flights to Mars and beyond. These are trips that could easily last two years, requiring every morsel of food to be selected carefully for maximum nutrition and efficiency. What the scientists found in their search was an amazing little grain that most Americans have never heard of: quinoa (pronounced keen-wah).

Their reasoning, as explained in a technical report, was simple.

"While no single food can supply all the essential life-sustaining nutrients," they wrote, "quinoa comes as close as any other in the plant or animal kingdom."

If the country's smartest minds are endorsing it, shouldn't you be eating it?

Quinoa may be overlooked in America—and most likely your very own household—but it has held legendary status for thousands of years in the Andes, where the locals use it for the energy they need to hike and live amid some of the world's most treacherous mountains. Although technically a seed, quinoa functions like a grain and is used as one. To the Incas, it was sacred. They called it *chisaya mama*, for "mother of all grains."

This preeminent status should have carried over to the rest of the world, but when the Spanish conquistador Francisco Pizarro and his men conquered the Incan empire in 1532, they shunned it, casting quinoa aside as a food for peasants and even razing many of the fields where it was grown. Instead Pizarro and his men chose to stock their ships with two crops—corn and potatoes—that shot to fame when they were taken to Europe a short time later.

Pizarro, who ruled with an iron fist and was eventually assassinated in an uprising in Lima in 1541, made more than a few blunders during his short time in Peru. Rejecting quinoa may have been the first.

But in his defense, there was no way he could have known what we know today. Myriad studies confirm it: quinoa is easily one of the world's healthiest foods.

Quinoa is extremely high in protein—up there with meat and dairy products—which by itself is very unusual for a food that comes from plants. It contains more protein and fewer carbs than wheat, rye, rice, or oats. Think about it this way: One cup of quinoa is packed with about as much protein as four eggs. And on top of that, the protein in quinoa is what nutritionists call "complete," meaning it contains all the essential amino acids, including lysine, which is critical to tissue growth and repair. As any vegetarian who struggles to get enough protein in his or her diet knows, it's hard to find a stat like that outside of the animal kingdom. It's a wonder these little grains don't come with skin and bones!

But protein is only the beginning of quinoa's nutritional story. Quinoa has a mineral content that blows barley, wheat, and other grains out of the water. One cup has more than half your daily requirement of iron, manganese, and magnesium (among other minerals). It's low in calories, and it's low in fat—and the fat that it does contain is the monounsaturated kind, which is good for your ticker anyway.

Then, of course, there's quinoa's fiber content, which is off the charts. According to the USDA, a single cup of uncooked quinoa contains about 12 grams of fiber, triple what you'd find in a lot of other grains. The average American adult—on a 2,000-calorie-a-day diet—needs about 25 grams of fiber. Eat two cups of quinoa a day and you're pretty much there.

With all of this going for it, it's no surprise that making quinoa a regular part of your diet has been shown to make you healthier. Epidemiological studies of tens of thousands of people over the years have shown that those who eat a daily bowl of quinoa or another high-fiber grain have lower rates of heart disease, type II diabetes, obesity, breast cancer, and premature death.

And if, after all of this, you're still not won over, there's the fact that quinoa is just darn tasty. Its soft texture and nutty flavor are reminiscent of couscous, only better.

When I brought quinoa to Dave and explained the science behind it, he was instantly sold. But I had to concede that I hadn't the slightest clue how to prepare it, and I asked Dave to give me a little demo.

"Oh, it's easy," he said. "It's pretty much like cooking rice."

And that's when my cooking deficiencies were fully revealed. You see, I don't really know how to cook rice. My way of preparing rice, as for a lot of New Yorkers, involves picking up my cell phone and ordering it from the Thai restaurant across the street. And the last time that happened, it cost me five dollars: two for the small carton of brown rice, and three to tip the delivery guy.

Luckily, Dave doesn't fall into the same camp of cooking-impaired New Yorkers. That being said, his experience with quinoa was relatively limited before I brought it to his attention, and he quickly started to discover many surprising nuances of this wonder ingredient.

"This stuff doesn't absorb nearly as much liquid as I thought it would!" he said on one of the first occasions he cooked with it, throwing a few frustrated expletives in there for good measure. "And even the people that sell this stuff have it wrong with their directions on all of these packages—they say to cook this stuff in way too much [insert a few more expletives] liquid!"

With a little more distance from the subject, Dave can now reminisce more calmly about the process. As he explains it:

Working with quinoa was a real discovery for me. I had never taken the time to get really comfortable with the grain or explore its range of uses—and the range is just amazing! But I was shocked that the directions out there for cooking quinoa in a ratio of one part quinoa to two parts water are leading home cooks to turn out just one big soggy mess that makes incorporating it tastefully into dishes a lot more challenging.

Once I figured out the correct ratio and consistently got my quinoa coming out light and fluffy, I was on a roll and could barely be stopped. I couldn't believe how versatile this stuff is. I was certain I wouldn't be able to get a breakfast or a dessert out of these little buggers, and yet sure enough I got both! In fact there's really only one way that quinoa doesn't taste good, and that's raw. But I figured out if you want some quinoa crunch without the raw flavor, all you have to do is dry some cooked quinoa in the oven for a while, which is exactly what I do with the brittle at the end of this chapter.

If you're looking to add some new flavor and a jolt of good health to your diet—and let's face it, who isn't?—quinoa is the way to go. Don't make the same mistake as Pizarro. Fill your cart with this wonder food and bid adieu to lesser foods.

cooking quinoa dave's way

Raw, unprocessed quinoa is naturally coated with saponins, a substance that is bitter, difficult to digest, and makes for soapy cooking water, so quinoa has to be washed before it can be cooked. But today it is rare to find quinoa in the market that isn't washed. Many packages of quinoa will be marked "prewashed" or "rinsed," but even quinoa that you can buy in bulk is generally prewashed, so you can skip that step and go right to the cooking. If you're worried about it, though, give the quinoa a quick rinse anyway.

Now when it comes to cooking the quinoa, never go by the directions on the package. Most directions that you will come across say to cook the quinoa with water in a ratio of 1 part quinoa to 2 parts water. But this results in quinoa that is much too wet and soggy. Quinoa should have the texture of couscous—dry, light, and fluffy. To achieve this result, cook quinoa in a ratio of 1 part quinoa to only 1¼ parts water.

Combine the quinoa and water in a heavy-bottomed pot (to avoid browning or drying of quinoa on the bottom of the pot) and season with a couple pinches of salt. Bring the quinoa and water to a simmer, reduce the heat to its lowest setting, and cover the pot. Cook for 20 to 25 minutes, until the quinoa is dry, light, and can easily be fluffed with a fork. Fluff well and let sit, uncovered, for a few minutes before serving or using in a recipe.

Creamy Breakfast Oats and Quinoa

Why not start your day with one of the healthiest foods on earth? Adding some oats to the mix gives you the familiar flavor and creaminess of oatmeal alongside the interesting texture and nutritional value of quinoa. For the creamiest results, always use whole oats rather than the quick-cooking or instant kind. Top the cooked mixture with fresh fruit, raisins, nuts, or seeds. Research shows that eating high-fiber grains like quinoa (which have a very low glycemic index) for breakfast keeps your blood sugar levels in check, won't make you crash, and even makes everything else you eat throughout the day less fattening.   SERVES 2

1½ cups milk, soy milk, or rice milk

1 tablespoon honey

¼ teaspoon ground cinnamon

Pinch of salt

½ cup cooked quinoa (see page 101)

¾ cup whole oats

In a small saucepan, bring the milk, honey, cinnamon, and salt to a simmer over medium heat. Add the quinoa and oats, cover, and cook until the mixture is thick and creamy and the oats are tender, 7 to 10 minutes.

CINNAMON

In American homes, cinnamon is probably the best-loved denizen of the spice rack. But when it comes to actually putting it to use on a regular basis, most home cooks can think of only oatmeal raisin cookies and maybe a dash in their Sunday pancake mix.

Cinnamon doesn't need to be relegated to the occasional baking project, however. In other countries cinnamon is used across a range of sweet and savory dishes, and incorporating those international influences into your cooking repertoire will help you get more cinnamon into your daily diet.

In Morocco, cinnamon is a key component of the classic meat braises known as *tagines*, which interplay sweet and savory in an intricate dance. In Mexico, cinnamon is a central seasoning for classic moles and chilies. Take a page from Mexican cooking and flavor stews and chilies with a hint of cinnamon to add a touch of warmth and a slight nod toward sweets.

And, of course, when it comes to baking, there is no end to the ways in which you can incorporate cinnamon. Just shy of arriving at cinnamon fatigue, try to add cinnamon to cakes and cookies; there are very few desserts in which a dash of cinnamon isn't welcome.

But cinnamon's impact is double-barreled: it's been shown in studies to help control blood sugar, and according to research by the USDA, it's also extremely high in antioxidants.

You can incorporate it into your diet in the ways just mentioned, or an easier, and perhaps even simpler way of getting a little cinnamon into your life is to sprinkle it on your coffee or frappuccino (or whatever fancy coffee creation happens to be your addiction; hey, we've all got 'em!).

Quinoa and Chickpea Falafel

Most people are scared of frying at home—all the oil; all the heat; all the mess. But it's simple: if you want good falafel, you've gotta fry. Minimize all the side effects by using a small saucepan to fry in small batches. And sure, this isn't low-fat, but I use canola oil, so you can still call it healthy! Look for chickpea flour in the organic or health food section of the supermarket or at Middle Eastern markets. MAKES ABOUT 30 FALAFEL

2 cups chickpea flour

½ teaspoon ground cumin

2 tablespoons olive oil

2½ cups boiling water

2 cups cooked quinoa (see page 101)

3 garlic cloves

2 teaspoons kosher salt

¼ cup fresh parsley leaves, finely chopped

Juice of 1 lemon

1½ teaspoons black pepper

About 3 cups canola oil, for deep-frying

Combine the chickpea flour, cumin, olive oil, and boiling water in a large mixing bowl. Mix well with a fork until a homogenous paste forms. Let stand for a couple minutes. Add the remaining ingredients except the canola oil.

Heat the canola oil in a small to medium saucepan to between 350°F and 375°F.

Use 2 metal spoons to make roughly shaped falafel balls, about 2 tablespoons in size, and drop the balls right into the hot oil. Fry in batches of only 5 or 6 at a time to prevent the oil from bubbling over and to keep the oil temperature relatively stable. Fry the falafel until golden brown, about 5 minutes, and then drain on a paper towel–lined plate.

Stuff the falafel into whole wheat pita pockets filled with chopped tomatoes, tahini, thinly sliced cucumber, quick-pickled cabbage (page 148), and hot sauce.

Ratatouille and Quinoa

Ratatouille is nothing more than a thoughtful conglomeration of Mediterranean vegetables, but it is so satisfying and tasty that even the most staunch carnivore might not wonder where the beef went. SERVES 6

I large eggplant

2 tablespoons kosher salt

¼ cup canola oil

I small onion, halved lengthwise and sliced crosswise about ⅛ inch thick

I large zucchini, halved lengthwise and thinly sliced crosswise about ¼ inch thick

I large yellow squash, halved lengthwise and thinly sliced crosswise about ¼ inch thick

4 garlic cloves, thinly sliced

3 large plum tomatoes, roughly chopped

¼ teaspoon hot red pepper flakes

I teaspoon dried basil

½ teaspoon dried marjoram

½ teaspoon dried thyme

2 tablespoons olive oil

4 cups cooked quinoa (see page 101)

Salt and freshly ground black pepper

Trim the ends off the eggplant and slice it lengthwise 1 inch thick. Stack the slices and cut them into 1-inch cubes. Place the cubes in a strainer over a large bowl, toss with the kosher salt, and let stand for a couple of hours at room temperature.

Heat the canola oil in a large skillet over high heat. Toss in the eggplant, onion, zucchini, and yellow squash. Reduce the heat to medium-high and cook, partially covered, stirring often, until the vegetables have softened, about 10 minutes.

Add the garlic, tomatoes, and herbs and cook, partially covered, until the mixture is thick and the vegetables are soft, about 10 minutes longer.

Remove from the heat, stir in the olive oil and the cooked quinoa.

Season with salt and pepper to taste.

Stewy Chipotle Black Beans over Quinoa

A couple of smoky chipotle peppers go a long way in this dish. In combination with the black beans and quinoa, this is a full meal in and of itself. Adding plenty of lime juice and freshly chopped cilantro makes a world of difference. SERVES 6

---

3 tablespoons canola or olive oil

I medium red onion, halved lengthwise and thinly sliced crosswise

2 canned chipotles packed in adobo, plus 2 tablespoons sauce

Two 15-ounce cans black beans, rinsed

2 cups chicken stock

3 garlic cloves, finely chopped

Juice of I lime

Sugar

Salt and freshly ground black pepper

I small bunch of fresh cilantro, tough stems removed, finely chopped

3 cups cooked quinoa (see page 101)

Heat the oil in a large saucepan or skillet over medium-high heat. Add the onion and cook until softened but still red, about 5 minutes. Finely chop the chipotles and add them to the onion, along with the adobo sauce, black beans, stock, garlic, and lime juice. Bring to a simmer, reduce the heat to medium, and cook, stirring often, for 15 to 20 minutes, until it is thickened and slightly reduced. Season with sugar, salt, and pepper to taste and finish with the chopped cilantro. Serve over the hot quinoa.

quinoa and life expectancy

Add a small bowl of quinoa to your daily diet and you may extend your expiration date. You don't have to look far to find the evidence.

In a groundbreaking 2004 report, scientists at the University of Minnesota compared the diets of more than 330,000 men and women in the United States and Europe, looking specifically at the amount of fiber they consumed on a daily basis over a period of six to ten years. The results leaned heavily in favor of the people who ate lots of quinoa and other high-fiber grains: those who did suffered the lowest rates of disease.

In fact, for every 10 grams of fiber the subjects added to their daily diets, they experienced a 10 percent reduction in their risk of suffering a coronary event. A cup of quinoa contains at least 12 grams of fiber. Make it two and you have at least a 20 percent reduction right there.

Add to that all of the other benefits linked to a high fiber intake—lower rates of cancer, type II diabetes, stroke, and high blood pressure—and there's no excuse not to add a bowl of quinoa to your day.

Warm Balsamic and Cucumber Quinoa Salad

This was the very first dish that I made for this chapter, and Anahad loved it so much he couldn't find anything to change. So I didn't. It is a very simple, fresh warm "salad." Plenty of balsamic vinegar and lots of fresh herbs make the dish a standout. SERVES 6

4 cups cooked quinoa (see page 101)

Leaves from 1 small bunch of fresh parsley, finely chopped

Leaves from 1 small bunch of fresh mint, finely chopped

2 large Persian or Israeli cucumbers, quartered lengthwise and thinly sliced (about 1 cup)

¼ cup olive oil

1 medium red onion, finely chopped

⅓ cup balsamic vinegar

Salt and freshly ground black pepper

Combine the quinoa, parsley, mint, and cucumbers in a large bowl and set aside.

Heat the oil in a small skillet over medium-high heat. Add the onion and sauté until it just begins to soften, about 3 minutes. Add the vinegar and cook until the mixture has thickened, about 5 minutes longer. Remove from the heat and toss with the quinoa mixture.

Quinoa-Stuffed Red Peppers

These Spanish-inspired stuffed peppers have all the makings of a full meal in one neat package. A side salad is all you need. Dried chorizo isn't typically considered a "health food," but much of the fat from the meat has been aged out, and because the sausage is so flavorful, only a small amount is needed to impart flavor to the quinoa. SERVES 6

¼ cup olive oil, plus more for rubbing the peppers

3 ounces dried chorizo, roughly chopped (about ½ cup)

1 large onion, halved lengthwise and thinly sliced crosswise

1 large green bell pepper, diced

2 garlic cloves, minced or pressed

1 teaspoon smoked paprika

Salt and freshly ground black pepper

4 cups cooked quinoa (see page 101)

6 large red bell peppers

Preheat the oven to 375°F.

Heat the olive oil in a large skillet over medium-high heat. Add the chorizo, onion, and green pepper and cook, stirring frequently, until the vegetables are soft and tender, about 10 minutes. Add the garlic and smoked paprika, season with salt and pepper to taste, and cook for 5 minutes longer. Stir in the cooked quinoa until fully incorporated and remove from the heat.

Slice the tops off the peppers about ½ inch from the stem so you make little pepper caps. Core and seed the peppers; then rub generously with olive oil. Fully stuff each pepper with the quinoa mixture, replace the peppers' caps, and place in a 9 × 13-inch baking dish.

Bake for 35 minutes, until the peppers have softened and start to take on a little color.

Shrimp and Quinoa Cakes with Gumbo Filé Sauce

When I started working on this chapter, I had just returned from a trip to New Orleans, where I had fallen in love with shrimp gumbo. So I knew I had to fit shrimp gumbo into this chapter. The absence of butter and the presence of quinoa along with all the fresh ingredients in this recipe create a nutritional feast. SERVES 6

For the Gumbo:

3 tablespoons canola oil

2 tablespoons all-purpose flour

1 large green bell pepper, roughly chopped

2 celery stalks, thinly sliced

1 large yellow onion, finely diced

1 teaspoon hot red pepper flakes

2 cups shrimp or seafood stock

2 cups chopped canned tomatoes

3 garlic cloves, minced

1 to 2 tablespoons filé powder, to taste

2 teaspoons Worcestershire sauce

Salt and freshly ground black pepper

For the Shrimp Cakes:

1 pound medium shrimp, peeled and deveined

3 tablespoons finely chopped fresh parsley leaves, plus more for garnish

2 cups cooked quinoa (see page 101)

1 teaspoon dry mustard

1 teaspoon ground coriander

1 teaspoon sweet paprika

Juice of ½ lemon

1 large shallot, minced

¼ cup canola oil, plus more for frying

2 egg whites, lightly beaten

Salt and freshly ground black pepper

To make the gumbo, heat the oil and flour in a heavy-bottomed 6-quart pot or very large skillet over high heat, stirring constantly, until the flour turns a dark caramel color, about 5 minutes. Reduce the heat to medium-high and add the green pepper, celery, and onion. Cook the vegetables until they are nice and soft, about 10 minutes.

Add the red pepper flakes, stock, tomatoes, garlic, filé powder, and Worcestershire sauce, bring to a simmer, and cook for 30 minutes longer. Season with salt and pepper to taste. Keep warm over low heat while you make the shrimp cakes.

To make the shrimp cakes, roughly chop all but 6 shrimp. Combine the chopped shrimp with the parsley, quinoa, mustard, spices, lemon juice, shallot, ¼ cup canola oil, and egg whites in a large mixing bowl.

Heat a couple tablespoons of canola oil in a nonstick skillet over medium-high heat. Form the shrimp mixture into cakes about 4 inches in diameter and 1 inch thick. Fry the shrimp cakes until golden brown, about 3 minutes on each side. Cook in batches, adding more canola oil as necessary.

When the cakes have been cooked, quickly sauté the reserved whole shrimp for just a couple minutes, until perfectly cooked. Top each shrimp cake with a ladle of gumbo and a whole shrimp and garnish with chopped parsley.

quinoa and iron

Quinoa is not only prized for its massive protein content; it's also a great source of iron—containing nearly a single day's worth in just ½ cup.

But the type of iron it contains is nonheme, which, unlike the type of iron found in meat and animal products (called *heme*), is not as easily absorbed and digested. However, if you throw some vitamin C into the mix, suddenly quinoa's iron content becomes far more accessible.

That's why we've paired this mighty grain with red and green peppers, both of which are brimming with iron-enhancing vitamin C. We chose to give red center stage, in part because it contains three times more vitamin C than its green counterpart. But you're welcome to flip the order. Either way, you're guaranteed to get tons of flavor—and of course plenty of iron.

Chinese Chicken and Vegetable Stir-Fry over Quinoa

The trick to a stir-fry is getting the pan screaming hot so that when you add the chicken and the eggplant there's plenty of built-up heat to brown them evenly. SERVES 6

---

1 pound skinless, boneless chicken breast, cut into ½-inch strips

1 medium Japanese eggplant, ends trimmed and sliced about ½ inch thick

4 garlic cloves, very finely chopped

¼ cup soy sauce

1 teaspoon dark sesame oil

¼ cup canola oil

¼ cup dark brown sugar

3 tablespoons rice or white wine vinegar

½ teaspoon ground allspice

1 tablespoon finely grated fresh ginger

1 teaspoon hot red pepper flakes

1 cup fresh broccoli florets

1 red bell pepper, thinly sliced lengthwise

1 onion, halved lengthwise and thinly sliced crosswise

1 large carrot, thinly sliced

One 8-ounce can water chestnuts, drained

4 cups cooked quinoa (see page 101)

Combine the chicken, eggplant, garlic, soy sauce, sesame oil, canola oil, brown sugar, vinegar, allspice, ginger, and red pepper flakes in a large bowl or resealable plastic bag. Cover and marinate for at least 30 minutes or overnight. Bring to room temperature before cooking.

In a steamer basket or makeshift steamer, steam the broccoli, bell pepper, onion, and carrot until al dente. Heat a dry cast-iron or stainless-steel skillet or wok over high heat for about 4 minutes. Sauté the marinated ingredients until the chicken is cooked through, about 5 minutes. Toss in the steamed veggies and water chestnuts and cook for a couple minutes longer to heat through. Serve over the cooked quinoa.

Linguine and Quinoa Meatballs with Tangy Tomato Sauce

Traditional meatballs depend on bread to give them a light body, but I thought some cooked quinoa could also fit the bill and add an extra protein punch while we're at it. Turns out, the quinoa works like a charm and the texture, while different from an Italian grandmother's, is quite wonderful in its own right. SERVES 6

For the Sauce:

¼ cup olive oil

I large onion, finely chopped

3 celery stalks, halved lengthwise and thinly sliced crosswise

I large carrot, quartered lengthwise and thinly sliced crosswise

I teaspoon hot red pepper flakes

One 28-ounce can tomatoes, chopped, with juices

4 garlic cloves, minced

I tablespoon balsamic vinegar

Salt and freshly ground black pepper

For the Meatballs:

3 tablespoons canola oil

I small onion, finely chopped

I pound lean ground beef

1½ cups cooked quinoa (see page 101)

½ cup finely grated Parmesan cheese

I egg

3 tablespoons fresh parsley leaves, very finely chopped

½ teaspoon salt

¾ teaspoon freshly ground black pepper

I pound linguine

I large handful fresh basil leaves

To make the sauce, heat the olive oil in a large pot over medium heat. Add the onion, celery, carrot, and red pepper flakes and cook until tender, 10 to 15 minutes. Add the tomatoes, garlic, and vinegar and simmer for 20 minutes longer. Season with salt and pepper to taste and set aside to keep warm.

To make the meatballs, preheat the oven to 425°F. Heat the canola oil in a small skillet over medium heat. Add the onion and cook, partially covered, until very soft, about 10 minutes. Remove from the heat and set aside to cool.

In a large mixing bowl, combine the beef, quinoa, Parmesan, egg, parsley, salt, pepper, and cooled onions. Stir until a smooth, homogenous mixture has formed.

Roll the meat mixture into 2-inch balls and set them on an aluminum foil–lined baking sheet in neat rows. Bake for 20 to 25 minutes, until nicely browned but still soft to the touch.

In a large pot of boiling water, cook the linguine al dente. Serve the pasta with some meatballs and the sauce and top with a sprinkling of torn basil leaves.

Toasted Quinoa and Nut Brittle

If you're going to eat candy, it might as well be of the redemptive sort. Some dry, toasted quinoa added to a traditional nut brittle makes this a nutritionally complete snack. After I made the first batch, Anahad and I went on a hard-hitting ski trip, and we stuffed a big bag of the brittle into our backpacks. It kept us fueled on the slopes the whole week.

¾ cup cooked quinoa (see page 101)

⅓ cup shelled raw sunflower seeds

⅓ cup hulled white sesame seeds

½ cup whole raw almonds, finely chopped (easiest in a food processor)

Canola oil for greasing

2 cups sugar

3 tablespoons honey

1 tablespoon butter

Preheat the oven to 300°F.

Spread the quinoa on a foil-lined baking sheet. Bake the quinoa about 30 minutes, until completely dry and toasted to golden brown. Transfer the toasted quinoa to a large mixing bowl and combine with the sunflower seeds, sesame seeds, and almonds.

Line the same baking sheet again with foil and grease it well with canola oil.

Use the canola oil to grease a large stainless-steel or Pyrex mixing bowl very well.

In a heavy-bottomed saucepan, combine the sugar, ½ cup water, and the honey and cook over medium-high heat until the mixture is bubbly and turns a very light amber color (for reference, this is 320°F on a candy thermometer). Swirl in the butter and immediately pour the mixture into the greased mixing bowl.

Work quickly to stir in the nut and quinoa mixture and then immediately pour the mixture onto the greased, foil-lined baking sheet. Use a metal spatula to press the mixture down into an even layer about ¾ inch thick.

Allow to cool fully and then break into snack-size pieces.

Note: Do not allow the mixture to harden on any cooking utensils or it will be difficult to remove.

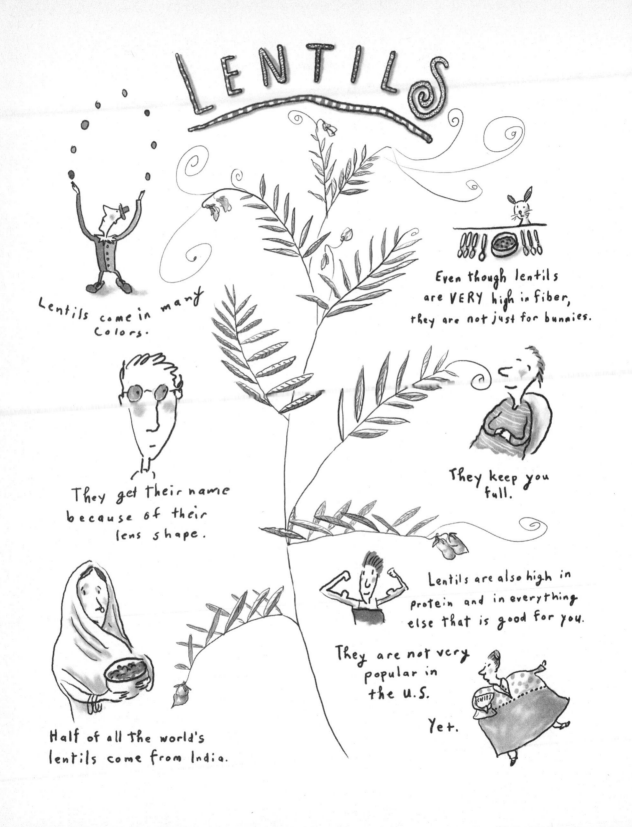

6

LENTILS

Why does fiber have such a bad rep?

Mentioning the word around most people conjures up thoughts of rabbit food and the FiberCon in Grandpa's medicine cabinet. It's not so much that fiber is hated as it is unloved. Sadly for many Americans, fiber has become more of a punch line than a part of the daily diet, a food so underappreciated that one of the world's highest-fiber foods needed a name change just to improve its image.

Take a walk through your local grocery store and you'll notice many packages previously labeled "prunes" now say "dried plums" instead. Fiber is no longer their main selling point; the packages have been slapped with statements about antioxidant content instead. Chalk that up to a $10 million makeover courtesy of the prune industry, which discovered in surveys that people were so averse to prunes and their fibrous image that if given the choice they would choose a dried plum over a prune—even though they are *exactly* the same. Fiber, it seems, is dismissed as food for old folks.

All of this is truly a shame, because the science on fiber is clear: it lowers cholesterol, reduces heart disease, and decreases the risk of overweight and diabetes.

American adults are supposed to eat a *minimum* of 20 to 35 grams of fiber a day. And yet studies consistently show that the average American adult eats only a fraction of that, somewhere between 12 and 18 grams a day. Children eat even less, getting only about a quarter of their recommended fiber intake. With statistics like that, it's no shock that the National Fiber Council found in 2007 that 88 percent of Americans surveyed had no idea how much fiber they should be eating and less than 50 percent even made a habit of checking food labels for fiber content.

Most weren't even sure what foods they could find fiber in: about 60 percent thought meat was a source of fiber. (Wrong.)

Americans have long been hooked on what scientists call a "high-calorie, low-fiber" Western diet. Is it any surprise then that one-third of adults are obese, one in five children is overweight, and heart disease is the number one killer of both men and women in America?

Isn't it about time that we finally flip that trend around? Fortunately for you, there's a way to get all the fiber you need without resorting to prune juice or your granddad's bottle of Metamucil. In supermarkets everywhere, there already exists a delicious, satisfying, and time-tested, though oft-overlooked, option.

We're talking about the humble lentil.

We know what you're thinking. *Lentils?* Yes, lentils. Chances are, you've never cooked a batch, and probably have never had a hearty meal in which lentils played a starring role in a restaurant either. Few people, even the most seasoned chefs, have any inclination to give this disk-shaped delicacy much of a chance.

But this could be your food awakening. The lentil's nutrient profile alone—high fiber, high protein, zero cholesterol, and nearly nonexistent fat—should, at the very least, persuade you to take a closer look.

These earthy legumes may seem tiny and meager, but the lentil is no ordinary bean. Each is a model of nutritional efficiency. Lentils are one of the highest-fiber foods on the planet, and second only to split peas among legumes. A single cup, cooked, is packed with about 16 grams of fiber, or 63 percent of the daily recommended value, and all of that won't run you more than a measly 25 cents!

Lentils aren't just your run-of-the-mill fiber-containing food: they're a double-barreled source. They are packed with soluble fiber, the kind of fiber that helps manage blood sugar (a boon for diabetics in particular) and that lowers your cholesterol by forming a gel-like substance that seeks out the bad kind of cholesterol, LDL cholesterol, and removes it from the body.

Lentils also boast insoluble fiber, better known as nature's scrub brush. Insoluble fiber passes through the body undigested, promoting regularity as it journeys through your system, speeding the movement of potentially toxic substances along the way, which may lower the risk of colon cancer and other diseases.

On a more practical level, the fiber in lentils keeps you full. Studies have shown that doubling the amount of fiber you eat can increase satiety and help regulate glucose and insulin. This may explain why studies have found that people who eat more fiber consistently gain less weight over the years than those who don't. In other words, eat a solid meal with lentils and the odds of ending up with your head back in the refrigerator an hour later fall sharply.

But there's even more reason to show lentils some love. Besides being loaded with fiber and a slew of minerals and vitamins—from folate to potassium and B vitamins—lentils are chock-full of two other nutritional jewels: protein and iron. At 18 grams per cup, lentils have more protein than almost any other plant source, just behind soybeans. And one cup provides 35 percent of your daily value of iron. Believe it or not, that's about the same as ground beef!

Why is this so significant? Because studies have consistently shown that a high intake of red meat might be hazardous to your health. In one large study financed by the National Cancer Institute in 2009, for example, scientists followed a half a million people over age fifty for a decade and found that those who ate the most red meat were most likely to die from cancer, heart diseases, and other causes during the study period, while those who ate the least were least likely to croak. Of course, the study was observational—meaning it didn't show a direct cause-and-effect relationship—and it's certainly not the final word on the matter. But the take-home message was that cutting back on red meat, even if only by a little, might be a good idea.

In fact, lentils have long been considered the ground beef of India, where half of the world's lentils are produced. Many vegetarians in India meet their nutrient needs by turning to lentils, which form a complete protein with all the essential amino acids when mixed with rice or another grain. But lentils were famous outside of India long ago. Lentils have been prized by cultures across the planet dating back to ancient times. They may have even been one of the first crops cultivated thousands of years ago in the Near East. Evidence of lentils being prepared as food as far back as ten thousand years ago has turned up along the banks of the Euphrates River in what today is northern Syria. And archaeologists have found lentils in Egyptian tombs, so not only were lentils not shunned, they were considered food fit for kings and queens in the afterlife!

From the Middle East, lentils spread rapidly, turning up in ancient Greece, India, China, and Babylon—and even making a cameo in the Bible. In Genesis, Esau, the oldest son of Isaac and Rebekah, finds his younger brother Jacob cooking a lentil stew after Esau has spent a long day in the fields. Famished, Esau begs for a bowl of the simmering lentils, eventually agreeing to trade his birthright as oldest son to Jacob for one hearty bowl. Now those must have been some darn good lentils!

And yet, despite such celebrated history, lentils remain underappreciated and underutilized here in the United States. This may simply be an issue of a knowledge gap. In the vegetarian household I grew up in, lentils were always part of our meals, from soups to small snacks, so I was many times more familiar with lentils than the average American. But it was only when I started hanging around a chef that I learned how truly versatile and flavorful this amazing little legume could be. Even after three decades of eating lentils, I was unprepared for the range and deliciousness of the recipes Dave was about to whip up. I figured there had to be some secret behind lentils, so I asked Dave to explain:

You know, there is no big secret to lentils. They are simple, humble little things, and really all they require is a bit of attention to bring out the best in them. Each member of the lentil family is a little different—they have different colors, different textures, and different cooking times—so it's all about picking the right lentil for the right dish. (See "Different Kinds of Lentils," page 126.)

Regardless of which lentil you pick, it's important to add the lentils at the right time in the cooking process so you wind up with the flavor and texture that you are going for. Obviously, with these recipes I've done that work for you, so all that's required is following the directions. But once you become familiar with the little nuances of each lentil, the door to a life of lentil freestyling will open.

Playing around with all these lentils was not only fun but also eye-opening. I was amazed at how much range I could get out of one lentil. For example, for a salad I cooked brown lentils just al dente and strained them until dry so that the texture of each lentil remained intact. But then I cooked the same brown lentils in some rich chicken stock and aromatics, and I was able to replicate the flavor and texture of refried beans!

So I really gotta hand it to lentils. After working with them pretty intensely, I can understand why they've been revered and loved all over the world for thousands of years. Give the following recipes a whirl, and pretty soon lentils may just have you willing to offer up your birthright!

Red Lentil and Red Pepper Soup

Red lentils break down more quickly and thoroughly than the darker variety of lentils, which make them a good choice for soups. You could puree the soup after adding the lentils, but I think it is more interesting to leave the texture as is. The bright color of the soup makes for a nice presentation, and while it can be served either cold or hot, I prefer it hot. SERVES 8

¼ cup olive oil

1 large leek, ends and tough green leaves trimmed, halved lengthwise, and thinly sliced

2 red bell peppers, finely chopped (about 2 cups)

1 quart chicken stock

1 cup dried red lentils

1 tablespoon balsamic vinegar

Salt and freshly ground black pepper

Heat the olive oil in a 6-quart pot over medium heat. Add the leek and peppers and cook, partially covered, until soft, about 10 minutes. Add the chicken stock and 2 cups water and simmer for 30 minutes. Remove from the heat and puree with an immersion blender. Return the soup to the heat, add the lentils, and cook for another 25 minutes, until the lentils are soft and broken down. Stir in the vinegar and season with salt and pepper to taste.

Brown Lentil Salad with Radicchio and Feta

While the ingredients of this salad are quite hearty, the effect of the ensemble is actually rather light and refreshing. I love the slight bitterness of the radicchio; its leaves are so robust that leftovers of the salad hold up well in the refrigerator, even up to two days later. SERVES 4

I cup dried brown lentils

¼ cup red wine vinegar

¼ cup canola oil

I tablespoon whole-grain mustard

I shallot, minced

I small head of radicchio, cored and roughly chopped

2 Persian or Israeli seedless cucumbers, ends trimmed, cut into ½-inch cubes

Leaves from I small bunch of fresh mint, roughly chopped

4 ounces imported feta, crumbled

Salt and freshly ground black pepper

Cook the lentils in 3 or 4 cups of salted boiling water until cooked through but still slightly firm, about 20 minutes. Drain and rinse under cold water to stop the lentils from cooking further. Set the lentils aside in the strainer to continue to dry.

Whisk together the vinegar, oil, mustard, and shallot.

Toss the dry lentils with the dressing, radicchio, cucumbers, mint, and feta. Season with salt and pepper to taste just before serving.

different kinds of lentils

There are dozens of varieties of lentils, and each one has its own unique flavor, appearance, and cooking nuances.

The most common lentils on American supermarket shelves are green and brown lentils, but with just a little more searching you should easily be able to find French lentils, red lentils, yellow lentils, and even black "beluga" lentils.

In general, the darker the lentil, the stronger the taste and the better able it is to stand up to the cooking process. Light-colored lentils, like red, yellow, and green, are mild in flavor and start to break down into a mushy consistency after just 20 minutes or so of cooking. French lentils, brown lentils, and black lentils, however, will hold their shape and their flavor for nearly twice as long as that, but they aren't nearly as creamy in texture.

When making a soup or a stew, you'll want the lentils to break down and turn a bit mushy, which is why you should reach for red, yellow, or green lentils. But when you want the firm, nutty texture of a lentil to come through, in a braised dish or a salad, opt for brown or French lentils.

The following table is a useful guide to cooking lentils.

Lentil Variety	Characteristics	Cooking Time	Uses
Red	Small to medium disks. Red, pink, and orange hues. Breaks down easily over the cooking process with a lightly creamy texture.	20–25 minutes	Soups, stews, dals, etc.
Yellow	Medium to large disks. Bright yellow color. Breaks down easily over the cooking process but not particularly creamy.	20–25 minutes	Soups, stews, dals, etc.
Green	Medium to large disks. Dull green color. Breaks down easily. Creamy texture.	25–30 minutes	Soups, stews, dips
Brown	Variety of sizes. The smaller the size, the firmer the texture. Light brown to dark brown color. Maintains shape well over the cooking process but will turn mushy if overcooked. Nutty flavor.	25–30 minutes	Salads, braises, dals, thick beanlike dishes
French	Small, dark green disks. Rich, peppery, nutty flavor. Firm texture and maintains shape very well over the cooking process.	35–50 minutes, depending on application	Salads, braises, hearty sides
Black	Small, rounder lentils. Firm texture, less assertive flavor. Maintains shape and color over the cooking process.	35–45 minutes, depending on application	Salads, braises, hearty sides

Red Lentil Dal with Cilantro and Yogurt

This is a flavor-packed Indian-inspired way to get your lentil quota for the day. SERVES 8

2 teaspoons ground coriander

2 teaspoons ground turmeric

2 teaspoons ground cumin

2 teaspoons ground cloves

2 teaspoons ground cardamom

1 teaspoon ground cinnamon

2 small dashes of cayenne

1 teaspoon salt

½ teaspoon freshly ground black pepper

¼ cup canola oil

2 medium onions, finely chopped

One 2-inch piece of fresh ginger, finely grated (about 1 heaping tablespoon)

2 cups cored and finely chopped plum tomatoes (about 5)

1½ cups dried red lentils

3 cups vegetable or chicken stock

Juice of ½ lemon

1 small bunch of fresh cilantro, roughly chopped

About 1 cup thick Greek-style yogurt

Stir together the spices, salt, and pepper in a small bowl.

Heat the oil in a large skillet over medium heat, add the onions, and cook, partially covered, stirring often, until they soften, about 5 minutes. Stir in the spice mixture and cook for a couple minutes longer. Stir in the ginger and tomatoes and cook, partially covered, until the tomatoes have softened, about 5 minutes. Stir in the lentils and stock and bring to a simmer.

Reduce the heat to low, cover, and cook until the lentils are soft and the mixture is thick, 20 to 25 minutes. Remove from the heat and stir in the lemon juice and cilantro.

Ladle into bowls and top with a couple good dollops of yogurt.

Lentil "Hummus"

The lentils are still hot when I use them in this recipe, resulting in a warm dip or spread that may even be better than the chickpea version. I like to serve this with crudités or with whole wheat pita loaves, cut into sixths and toasted in a 350°F oven for about 10 minutes. SERVES 6 TO 8

I cup dried green lentils

2 garlic cloves, peeled

2 tablespoons unsalted tahini

Juice of I lemon

½ teaspoon ground cumin

I teaspoon sweet paprika, plus more for garnish

I handful fresh parsley leaves

½ cup olive oil, plus more for garnish

Salt and freshly ground black pepper

Cook the lentils in a quart of salted boiling water until soft but not falling apart, no more than 20 minutes. Strain the lentils and add them to a food processor along with the garlic, tahini, lemon juice, cumin, 1 teaspoon paprika, parsley, and ½ cup olive oil. Process until completely smooth. Season with salt and pepper to taste, then spoon into a large, shallow bowl. Finish with a dash of paprika and a good drizzle of olive oil.

TURMERIC

Turmeric flies under the radar of most people in this country. Although it is one of the most popular and most widely consumed spices in our diet, you would be hard-pressed to find Americans who know when they are even eating the stuff.

Believe it or not, though, turmeric is in pretty much every curry powder and every bottle of commercial ballpark-style mustard you have ever bought. It is used to flavor a wide range of dishes, from rice stir-fries to sweet custards.

However you end up incorporating it, be sure to pat yourself on the back: turmeric is widely believed by scientists to help fight inflammation and lower the risk of Alzheimer's and some forms of cancer.

In the United States, turmeric is sold in the spice aisle in a ground, powdered form derived from the turmeric root, and it is instantly recognizable for its dark orange-yellow hue. Turmeric's colorant abilities are so strong that it is even used to dye cloth in some parts of the world. It is the same potent characteristic that makes it so valuable to cooks across the globe. Often called the "poor man's saffron," turmeric is used to impart a golden hue to traditional dishes, such as paella, when saffron is unavailable or simply too expensive.

That's not to say that turmeric isn't appreciated for its flavor, but too much turmeric will leave your dishes tasting extremely earthy and bitter. When used judiciously, on the other hand, it can add a hint of warmth and complexity to many a dish.

I obviously depend on turmeric whenever I use curry powder, but I also will incorporate it in simpler ways, like putting a teaspoon of turmeric into the salted boiling water for a pot of rice.

Roasted Salmon over French Lentils, Tomatoes, and Fennel

French green lentils are probably the most venerated of the lentils you will find at your supermarket—and for good reason. They have a robust, earthy flavor and a toothsome quality that few other lentil varieties possess. They are also very versatile, as they can stand up to heavy meat preparations. But in this recipe they add some interesting depth to a lighter preparation. SERVES 6

¼ cup olive oil

I large onion, thinly sliced lengthwise

I small fennel bulb, cored, ends trimmed, and thinly sliced lengthwise

I pound fresh plum tomatoes, cored and roughly chopped (about 2 cups)

½ teaspoon dried marjoram

½ teaspoon dried thyme

½ cup dry white wine

I quart chicken stock

1½ cups French green lentils (*lentilles du Puy*)

2 garlic cloves, minced

Salt and freshly ground black pepper

6 small salmon fillets, about 4 ounces each

¼ cup olive oil

Juice of ½ lemon

Lemon wedges, for serving

Preheat the oven to 400°F.

Combine the oil, onion, fennel, tomatoes, marjoram, and thyme in a large saucepan over medium heat and cook, partially covered, stirring frequently, until the fennel is soft, about 15 minutes. Add the wine and cook, uncovered, for 5 minutes longer. Add the stock, bring to a simmer, and stir in the lentils and garlic. Cook until the lentils are tender and the mixture has thickened, about 30 minutes longer. Season with salt and pepper to taste and keep warm.

Toss the salmon fillets with the olive oil, lemon juice, and salt and pepper to taste. Place the fillets on a foil-lined baking sheet and roast until the fish is medium, about 10 minutes.

Spoon the lentils into large, shallow bowls and top with the roasted salmon. Serve with the lemon wedges.

Giant Chicken and "Refried" Lentil Quesadillas

Anahad is a lover of spicy, boldy flavored Mexican food, so this recipe ranks as one of his favorites. The lentils stand in for the traditional beans, but I prepare them in very much the same way. The dish turned out so well that I may never go back. You will likely have some extra salsa, but that's good news; it makes for a fantastic dip for chips, and it will keep for up to a week in the refrigerator. SERVES 8

For the Refried Lentils:

2 tablespoons canola oil

1 large onion, finely chopped

1 tablespoon chili powder

1 cup dried brown lentils

½ teaspoon Tabasco sauce

2 cups chicken stock

Salt

For the Salsa:

2 small onions, peeled and cut into eighths

1 pound plum tomatoes, cored and halved lengthwise

8 ounces tomatillos, husked and quartered

2 garlic cloves, smashed

About 3 chipotle chiles packed in adobo sauce

2 tablespoons canola oil

Salt

Juice of 2 limes

1 small bunch of fresh cilantro, tough stems removed

For the Quesadillas:

Four 8-inch whole wheat round wraps

1 rotisserie chicken, about 2 pounds, meat pulled from the bones and loosely shredded

8 ounces Monterey Jack cheese, finely grated (about 2 cups)

2 large avocados, pitted, peeled, and roughly chopped

Preheat the oven to 400°F.

To make the refried lentils, heat the oil in a saucepan over medium heat. Add the onion, and cook, partially covered, stirring often, until softened and starting to turn translucent, about 5 minutes. Stir in the chili powder and cook for a minute longer; then add the lentils, Tabasco sauce, and chicken stock. Bring the mixture to a simmer and cook, covered, until the lentils have turned soft and mushy and have the consistency of refried beans when stirred, about 30 to 35 minutes. Season with salt to taste and set aside.

To make the salsa, toss the onions, tomatoes, tomatillos, garlic, and chipotle chiles with the oil on a foil-lined baking sheet. Season with salt to taste and roast for about 20 minutes, until the vegetables are soft and juicy and the tomatoes have collapsed. Transfer the cooked vegetables to a food processor and process with the lime juice and cilantro until a smooth salsa forms.

To make the quesadillas, place 2 of the wraps on a large foil-lined baking sheet. Divide the lentils between them and spread them out smoothly. Divide the pulled chicken evenly between the wraps; then top each one with about ½ cup of the salsa and a good handful or so of the shredded cheese.

Close the quesadillas by covering with the remaining wraps and bake for 10 minutes, until the wraps begin to brown and the cheese has melted. Remove the wraps from the oven and top with the remaining salsa, chopped avocados, and remaining cheese. Bake for 5 minutes longer; then transfer to a large cutting board and cut each quesadilla into quarters.

lentils and glycemic index

Need another reason to love lentils? Here's one that comes down to two words: *glycemic index.*

You've probably heard that phrase thrown around a lot lately, but its meaning still isn't widely known.

It's simple, really: All carbs are not created equal.

Carbs are digested at different rates. Some carbs break down rapidly and almost immediately shoot glucose into the bloodstream, while others break down slowly and release glucose into the bloodstream more gradually. The glycemic index is a measure of just how quickly (or slowly) a certain food raises your blood sugar.

Why does this matter? Because studies suggest that frequent and regular intake of high–glycemic index foods can increase the risk of obesity, diabetes, and other chronic conditions. Some of the foods that have the highest index values (high is defined as anything with a value greater than 70) include the usual suspects: doughnuts and waffles (76), baguettes (95), sugary cereals (75 or above), and cookies (80 and above).

But lentils, you'll be happy to know, are exceptionally low on the list. Any food with a glycemic index of 55 or below is considered low. Green lentils have a measly GI value of 29. High in protein and fiber and low in bad carbs, there are lots of reasons to love lentils.

Lentil and Turkey Chili

This recipe makes *a lot* of chili. It is just the thing for a big, hearty, comfy meal with friends or family. SERVES 12

---

3 tablespoons canola oil

1 large onion, finely chopped

3 celery stalks, halved lengthwise and thinly sliced crosswise

2 ancho chiles, rinsed, patted dry, stems removed, and roughly chopped

2 pounds ground turkey, preferably white meat

Half 6-ounce can tomato paste

One 26-ounce can crushed tomatoes

1 quart chicken stock

One 12-ounce bottle lager beer

2 tablespoons chili powder

2 teaspoons ground cumin

½ teaspoon ground cloves

2 tablespoons cider vinegar

2 teaspoons Tabasco sauce, or more if desired

2 teaspoons Worcestershire sauce

3 tablespoons molasses

⅓ cup strong freshly brewed coffee

1½ cups dried brown or green lentils

Two 15-ounce cans kidney beans, drained and rinsed

Heat the oil in a large, heavy-bottomed pot over medium heat. Add the onion, celery, and ancho chiles and cook, stirring often, until the vegetables have softened, about 10 minutes. Add the turkey and cook, stirring consistently, until the meat has crumbled and cooked through, about 10 minutes. Add in the tomato paste and cook 5 minutes more.

Add the canned tomatoes, stock, beer, chili powder, cumin, cloves, vinegar, Tabasco, Worcestershire, molasses, and coffee. If the mixture looks too thick, pour in some water and bring to a simmer. Cook, partially covered, stirring often, for 1½ hours. Then add the lentils and kidney beans and cook for 1 hour longer.

Serve with condiments of your choice.

lentils and the environment

Lentils aren't just good for the body—they're good for the environment as well. According to climate scientists, roughly half of the greenhouse gas emissions stemming from our patterns of food consumption come from meat, even though beef, pork, and chicken account for less than 15 percent of what we eat. Beef alone produces a stunning 19 kilograms of carbon dioxide for every kilogram consumed (even grass-fed beef), and studies show that for every reduction in meat consumption in our diets, there is a corresponding decline in toxic effects on the environment.

That's where lentils come in. They are far more environmentally friendly. And with their high protein and iron content and their meaty texture, they make the perfect companion to red meat. Take a red meat recipe—like burgers, for example—and then cut the amount of beef roughly in half and swap in lentils. You'll keep the protein, iron, and hearty substance, while cutting back on the sodium, saturated fat, trans fat, calories, and cholesterol—not to mention all the greenhouse gas emissions. And on top of that, you add fiber and a slew of nutrients to your meat.

That's what we like to call a Better Burger.

The Better Burger

Broiling these burgers eliminates the need for any added fat, and the lentils make for a lighter texture without taking away from the flavor of the beef. Be sure to cook the lentils until they are very soft; otherwise they'll have trouble staying incorporated into the burger. SERVES 6

---

3 tablespoons canola oil

1 medium onion, finely chopped

1 pound lean ground beef

1 cup dried green lentils, cooked until very soft, as in lentil "hummus" (page 129)

1 large garlic clove, minced

2 tablespoons fresh parsley leaves, finely chopped

1 teaspoon Worcestershire sauce

1 tablespoon ketchup

1 teaspoon salt

½ teaspoon freshly ground black pepper

6 burger buns, preferably whole wheat

Preheat the broiler to high with the rack about 6 inches from the heat element.

Heat the oil in a large skillet over medium-high heat. Add the onion and cook, stirring often, until soft and translucent, about 7 minutes. Remove from the heat and set aside to cool.

In a large mixing bowl, combine the ground beef, cooked lentils, garlic, parsley, Worcestershire, ketchup, salt, and pepper. Stir in the cooked onion.

Form 6 patties, about 4 inches in diameter and 1 inch thick, and place them on a foil-lined baking sheet.

Broil the burgers until they reach the desired doneness, about 5 minutes per side for medium.

Top with sliced avocado, sliced onions, sliced vine-ripened tomatoes, butter lettuce, and any condiments of your choice.

Smoked Ham Hock and Green Lentil Stew

There are many different variations of ham hocks at the supermarket. Look for lean ones with a thick skin and the thinnest layer of fat between the meat and the skin. You don't need to add much salt to the dish, because salt has already been added to the ham hocks during the smoking process. SERVES 8

4 smoked ham hocks (about 1½ pounds total)

2 large carrots, finely chopped

1 large onion, finely chopped

3 celery stalks, finely chopped

2 large bay leaves

2 cups dried green lentils

Tabasco sauce

Salt and freshly ground black pepper

Combine the ham hocks, carrots, onion, celery, and bay leaves in a large stockpot. Add just enough cold water to cover all the ingredients and bring to a simmer over medium-high heat. Cover and simmer for 1 hour, until the meat of the ham hocks is very tender.

Remove the ham hocks from the cooking liquid, discard the skin and any fat, and pull the meat from the bones. Add the meat and the bones back to the cooking liquid, and add the lentils. Cook for 45 minutes longer, until the lentils are broken down and the mixture is thick. Season with Tabasco sauce and salt and pepper to taste.

CABBAGE

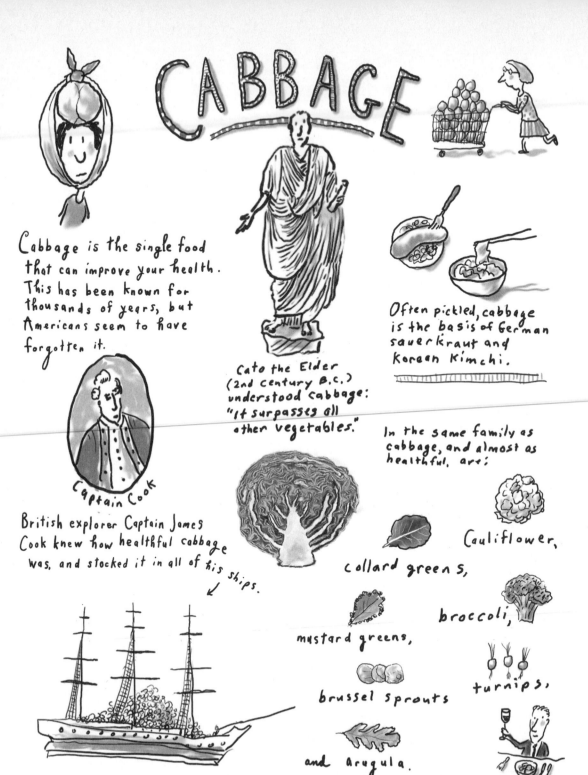

Cabbage is the single food that can improve your health. This has been known for thousands of years, but Americans seem to have forgotten it.

Cato the Elder (2nd century B.C.) understood cabbage: "It surpasses all other vegetables."

Often pickled, cabbage is the basis of German sauerkraut and Korean kimchi.

Captain Cook

British explorer Captain James Cook knew how healthful cabbage was, and stocked it in all of his ships.

In the same family as cabbage, and almost as healthful, are:

Cauliflower,

collard greens,

broccoli,

mustard greens,

brussel sprouts

turnips,

and arugula.

7

CABBAGE

Can a single food change your life?

Pose this question to Dorothy Pathak, a cancer researcher at Michigan State University, and her response is unwavering: absolutely. A Harvard-trained epidemiologist, Pathak has long been on the front lines of the effort to uncover how food and environment impact health, focusing in particular on ways to prevent cancer. In 1995 she moved to East Lansing to join the faculty at Michigan State, where she noticed something peculiar in two nearby cities, Chicago and Detroit. Both of these major cities have sizable Polish-American populations, and in both communities, separated by a lake and nearly three hundred miles, an unusual explosion of disease was unfolding.

In both cities, Polish women were being struck by high rates of breast cancer. What was particularly disturbing, Pathak noted, was that this seemed to be a local phenomenon. Women who immigrated to these cities quickly developed almost triple the risk of breast cancer when compared with their kin who stayed behind in the Old Country, putting them on a par with their American counterparts, among whom breast cancer is a leading killer.

Even more unusual was that Polish immigrants seemed to be alone in this pattern. Women who immigrated to the United States from countries like China and Japan did not see the same spikes in cancer; their risk generally remained the same as that of their kin back home.

Mystified, Pathak's thoughts turned to diet. At first, many in the scientific community resisted the idea that dietary changes could be responsible. But Pathak, who is Polish-American herself, launched a study in conjunction with the National Cancer Institute and said she quickly figured it out. The answer, she told me, was cabbage, a wonder vegetable widely known for its power to protect health.

In Poland, cabbage is a staple in the diet, served with nearly every meal. People there eat an estimated 30 pounds of the vegetable every year. But after examining the eating habits of Polish immigrants before and after they arrived in the United States, Pathak found that once they settled on American soil, their consumption of cabbage dropped significantly. This minor dietary tweak had a major result. Pathak found that women who stopped eating cabbage saw their risk of breast cancer soar. Those who continued to eat it at least three times a week saw their risk plummet. And women who had been "high consumers" of cabbage since adolescence had what essentially amounted to lifetime protection.

One food, it seemed, had the power to fend off cancer—but how?

At the University of Illinois, another team of scientists that was struck by the cancer rates among Polish immigrants in Chicago and Detroit also homed in on cabbage. The epidemiological evidence was already in. But to confirm it, they went to the lab, where they grew colonies of cancer cells and then exposed them to cabbage extracts. The scientists made sure to use small, realistic doses of extract—amounts that a person would get from eating normal amounts of the vegetable.

When the results came in, they were clear as day. The cabbage extract proved its mettle, throwing up a roadblock that caused the cancer cells to jam on their brakes. Eventually scientists discovered an entire slew of compounds in the extract that seemed capable of playing a role not only in breast cancer but also in several other forms of the disease—stomach, lung, and prostate cancer, among others—as well as heart disease, ulcers, Alzheimer's, gastrointestinal problems, and a variety of other conditions.

Of course, even the strongest studies offer no guarantees: there is no such thing as a food that doubles as a panacea. But eating cabbage does appear to be a surefire way to help safeguard your health; that much is clear.

To anyone familiar with the history of cabbage, this may come as little surprise: the vegetable has been prized for its medicinal properties for thousands of years.

Back then cabbage didn't look anything like the shiny red and green heads that you get in your supermarket today. In fact, the original wild cabbage plant didn't have a head at all. Instead it resembled something closer to kale. Of course there's a good reason for this: cabbage and kale are actually in the same family; they're so closely related, in fact, that they are essentially siblings.

It's a bit confusing, but both cabbage and kale—and many other of our most beloved and most widely consumed veggies—are part of a genus of plants known as *cruciferous vegetables*. The more colloquial name for this genus is simply "the cabbage family," and the family includes the likes of collard greens, broccoli, cauliflower, mustard greens, turnips, napa cabbage, and even arugula! Some of these are more closely related than others, but basically what happened was that humans harvested the cabbage plant and cultivated it different ways in different parts of the world, giving us the variety of cabbage relatives that we know today.

All of the descendants of the wild cabbage plant have healthful properties, but studies seem to home in on the subgroup of cruciferous veggies containing modern-day cabbage, whose health-giving powers seem to be particularly potent.

In the Mediterranean, where cabbage is believed to have originated, Cato the Elder, the famous statesman and agriculturalist also known as Cato the Wise, extolled cabbage as far back as the second century B.C., promoting it as a cure for everything from digestive problems to hangovers and liver disease.

"It is the cabbage which surpasses all other vegetables," he wrote. "What virtue and health-giving qualities it has."

As time progressed, that reputation followed cabbage as it spread throughout Europe. Pickled cabbage became a mainstay in Poland and Hungary, eventually finding its way to dinner tables in Scandinavia, where it was prized for its ability to survive the brutal winters. German sailors, apparently aware of its high vitamin C content, packed fermented cabbage on long trips, using it to ward off scurvy. Captain James Cook, the famed British explorer and navigator, noticed this in the late 1700s and became convinced of the medicinal powers of cabbage, insisting that British crews stock their ships with sauerkraut for long voyages.

Meanwhile, cabbage was enjoying fame in Asia as well, where it was widely prepared with little more than salt and water. By the twelfth century, it was common to add other spices to the dish. This more flavorful preparation exploded in popularity and remains today a staple of Asian cuisine, perhaps most notably in Korea, where it's known as *kimchi*.

Perhaps all these cultures relished these cabbage preparations simply for their bold taste rather than their potent health benefits, but today we know from studies that cabbage is plush with a unique set of nutrients that, despite their intimidating names, do their job of fighting off toxins with elegant precision.

Leading this list is something you can't help but love, sulforaphane. Forget trying to pronounce it. Just know that scientists at Johns Hopkins—led by Dr. Paul Talalay, a distinguished pharmacology professor—showed that it helps mobilize the immune system to gang up on carcinogens and other foreign intruders, sweeping them out of the body. That may explain why scientists have also found a decreased risk of prostate and lung cancers in high consumers of cabbage. The Hopkins scientists were so impressed by the compound, which is also found in broccoli and other cruciferous vegetables, that they developed a special technique allowing them to select seeds with the highest content so they could market them, with part of the proceeds going to research on cancer prevention.

And that's only one of a bunch of potent players that can be found in cabbage. One in particular—saddled with the unfortunate moniker of *indole-3-carbinol*—acts like a nutritional strongman. Most people know that estrogen plays a strong role in breast cancer. The reason is that when estrogen is broken down in the body, it can take one of two metabolic pathways: turning into either a compound that fuels tumors or a second one that is relatively inert and harmless. Indole-3-carbinol prefers the second pathway, because it aggressively pushes estrogen to take the more innocent route toward becoming inert.

Then there's cabbage's vitamin K content, which protects the joints and significantly lowers the risk of osteoarthritis. All it takes is a single serving of coleslaw to nearly meet the entire daily amount of vitamin K recommended by the USDA. Add to that the fact that those deceptively lean leaves are chock-full of vitamin C, vitamin

A, calcium, fiber, folate, and plenty of other nutrients—including even omega-3, which most people associate only with fish—and it's obvious why scientists have jumped on the cabbage bandwagon.

But the average American has yet to catch on: most people never eat cabbage unless it's dumped on a hot dog or served in a thimble-sized cup alongside a cheeseburger. Dr. Pathak, the epidemiologist, said that even she had fallen into this nutritional rut. Growing up in Poland, she ate cabbage all the time. When she moved to the United States in 1965, however, that quickly changed.

"I would say the amount of cabbage I ate actually almost dropped to zero, nil, when I moved here," she said.

She chalks that up to two things.

"One is I married a Hindu, an Indian, so my diet changed a lot," she says with a laugh. "And the second reason is that after we were married we moved to New Mexico. There aren't too many Polish stores that have cured sauerkraut like there are in Chicago and in Detroit."

But after her work on cancer and cabbage, she went back to her old ways. Now she whips up homemade coleslaw, using raspberry vinaigrette instead of mayonnaise, and she makes sure her nineteen-year-old daughter loads up on cabbage as well. A friend of Pathak's took to using leaves of cabbage instead of lettuce on the sandwiches she makes for her and her two teenage sons. Other people who learn about the cabbage-cancer link invariably come back to Pathak and say they've changed their habits as well.

"They come back to me, and they say, 'Guess what? We're eating more cabbage now!' or 'Today when I had my coleslaw, I was thinking of you,'" Pathak says. "It's not very difficult to adopt it within your diet—and it tastes good."

No one knows this better than Dave:

Pound for pound, dollar for dollar, I can't think of another ingredient that delivers more in the kitchen than cabbage. One small head of cabbage, which sets me back only a couple bucks, is enough for a huge bowl of a crisp summer slaw or a feast-sized one-pot meal.

Given my Eastern European heritage, I have a predetermined penchant for cabbage. I love it basically any way it's prepared, whether stewed, braised, shredded, or boiled. And thanks to Anahad, now I know that's great news for my health!

But really what I find most miraculous about cabbage is how, with the addition of heat, it transforms itself from something tough and slightly bitter into something so sweet and succulent, melding seamlessly into the flavors of the other ingredients in a dish. I suppose that is what makes it so loved in so many parts of the world, from Africa to Eastern Europe, giving me a great excuse to dabble in different ethnic cuisines with each head of cabbage I buy.

Stewed Red Cabbage, Red Onions, and Dried Cranberries

I fell in love with this sweet-and-sour preparation of red cabbage during my time in Germany, where the dish is served almost like a condiment alongside roasted meats. But it is also delicious on its own. Using dried cranberries isn't traditional, but I like what they add, and they certainly fit into the color scheme! SERVES 8

I small red cabbage, halved, cored, and sliced about ¼ inch thick

I large red onion, thinly sliced

I cup dried cranberries

⅓ cup turbinado or other raw sugar

¾ cup red wine vinegar

I cup chicken or vegetable stock

Salt to taste

Combine all the ingredients in a large pot and bring to a simmer over medium-high heat. Cover, reduce the heat to low, and cook, stirring from time to time, until the mixture is soft and thick, about 1 hour.

Pickled Cabbage and Onions

This is a good standby to have in the fridge or pantry to serve with sandwiches or roasted meats. The longer you let the jarred cabbage sit, the tastier it becomes. Also try it with my falafel (see page 104).

Also try it with my falafel (see page 104).

MAKES SIX 1-PINT JARS

I small head of green cabbage (1½ to 2 pounds), cored and cut into roughly 2-inch pieces

I large onion, halved and thinly sliced lengthwise

2 tablespoons kosher salt

3 cups white vinegar

2 tablespoons sugar

3 tablespoons pickling spice

4 bay leaves

Toss the cabbage and onion together with the salt in a large strainer or colander set over a big bowl. Cover with plastic wrap and let stand for several hours, tossing occasionally, until the cabbage has wilted down to less than half of its original volume. Divide the cabbage and onion combination among three 1-pint jars, packing loosely.

Bring the vinegar, 2 cups of water, sugar, and spice to a simmer in a small saucepan over medium-high heat. As soon as the mixture has reached a simmer, remove from the heat and pour into the cabbage-filled jars to fill them. Seal the lids and allow to cool before refrigerating.

Keeps up to 3 months in the refrigerator.

when to use which cabbage

While the differences between heads of cabbage may seem slight, they are actually quite individual, each offering a unique set of qualities in the kitchen.

Green cabbage, in its raw state, is pungent, slightly spicy, and tough. Mild, sweet tenderness must be coaxed out of it gently and slowly. Crisp spiciness can be just the right thing for a salad or a condiment, but otherwise some long, slow heat is in order, which makes soups, stews, and braises the best vehicles for this variety.

Red cabbage is prettier and sweeter than green cabbage, but when cooked it stands out boldly with its intense purple color and earthy sugars. This makes it a bit of a hard thing to pair, which is why we prefer it best on its own, as in the recipe for sweet stewed red cabbage (page 147). Keep in mind that when you're cooking red cabbage its color will fade rapidly in an alkaline environment, which is why adding vinegar or another acid to the mix is so important. One of the best things about cooked red cabbage is its vibrant color, so it's a shame to lose it.

Savoy cabbage is the prince among cabbages. Look closely at it and you may be reminded of intricately designed lace or an elaborate spiderweb. Its ribs are thin and flexible, and its leaves are tender and beautifully colored. Tender savoy cabbage requires less cooking time than its cousins, and it turns translucent when it's ready to be eaten. This makes it the perfect cabbage for incorporating into more refined dishes or when a pliable piece of cabbage is helpful, as in the recipe for stuffed cabbage on page 162. Because savoy cabbage is tender to begin with, it doesn't require long cooking times, which makes it a good choice for a faster preparation, like my linguine recipe on page 159.

Brussels Sprout Salad with Soy-Caramelized Shiitakes

Anahad is a regular at a restaurant here in New York City where they serve a very simple shaved Brussels sprout salad with shaved pecorino. This is my riff on that salad. I especially enjoy the contrast between the crunchy sliced sprouts and the soft, sweet shiitake mushrooms. After I cook the mushrooms, I don't let them cool completely, so the salad is just a touch warm when served. SERVES 4 TO 6

For the Salad:

6 ounces shiitake mushrooms, stems removed and caps sliced about ½ inch thick

2 tablespoons light soy sauce

2 tablespoons rice wine vinegar

2 tablespoons canola oil

1½ tablespoons dark brown sugar

½ teaspoon hot red pepper flakes

2 garlic cloves, thinly sliced

For the Dressing:

⅓ cup olive oil

⅓ cup fresh lemon juice (from about 1½ lemons)

Leaves from 4 fresh thyme sprigs

3 garlic cloves, smashed

1½ pounds Brussels sprouts, ends trimmed, halved lengthwise, and thinly sliced lengthwise

About 2 ounces pecorino cheese, shaved

Salt and freshly ground black pepper

In a resealable plastic bag, combine the shiitakes, soy, vinegar, oil, brown sugar, hot red pepper flakes, and garlic. Seal the bag and marinate for at least 30 minutes at room temperature and up to overnight in the refrigerator.

Transfer the mushrooms and marinade to a small skillet over medium-high heat. Cook the mushrooms, mixing often, until the liquid from the marinade and the mushrooms evaporates and the mushrooms darken in color, about 7 minutes. Remove from the heat and set aside to cool.

In a large mixing bowl, whisk together the dressing ingredients. Add the thinly sliced Brussels sprouts, followed by the cooked mushrooms, and toss well. Season with salt and pepper to taste (you shouldn't need much salt due to the soy sauce in the mushrooms). Arrange the salad on plates and garnish each serving with a couple good pinches of pecorino and more black pepper.

brussels sprouts

Much like broccoli, Brussels sprouts are a close relative of cabbage that deserve special mention.

The vegetable, named for its link to the capital of Belgium—Brussels—where it is believed to have originated, is rarely put to good use in American kitchens. Many children grow up despising the steamed Brussels sprouts that seem to be their only iteration in most households.

But Brussels sprouts are naturally crisp and crunchy, and the leaves are much thicker than plain old lettuce, making them perfect for exciting new salads with a twist.

They're also linked to great health. Like cabbage and broccoli, Brussels sprouts are high in certain antioxidants that have been shown in studies to help lower the risk of various cancers.

The sprouts are also high in vitamin A, which helps protect vision and bulk up the immune system, and folate, a crucial vitamin that helps reduce the risk of neurological conditions like Alzheimer's and dementia.

Since Brussels sprouts share a nutrient profile similar to that of cabbage, mixing them into your diet is a good way to get a little variety and still reap the benefits of cabbage. Just don't steam them and put them on a plate for your kids.

Cabbage, Cauliflower, and Potato Chowder

A hint of mustard and some flash-browned cabbage make this dish fit for a German beer garden, but it could also work equally well as the beginning to an elegant meal. SERVES 8

5 tablespoons canola oil

I large onion, finely chopped

2 russet potatoes (8 ounces each), peeled and cut into ½-inch cubes

½ head of green cabbage (about I pound), finely shredded, plus 2 cups for garnish

½ head of cauliflower (about I pound), cored and roughly chopped

I quart chicken or vegetable stock

2 tablespoons whole-grain mustard

Salt and freshly ground black pepper

Heat 3 tablespoons of the oil in a large, heavy-bottomed pot over medium heat. Add the onion and cook, partially covered, stirring often, until softened and translucent, about 5 minutes. Add one of the cubed potatoes, the ½ head of cabbage, cauliflower, chicken stock, and 1 quart of water, or as much as is needed to just cover all the ingredients. Bring to a simmer, reduce the heat to low, and cook until the cauliflower is so tender it falls apart at the slightest prodding of a fork, about 45 minutes.

Remove the pot from the heat and use an immersion blender to puree the soup. Then add the remaining cubed potato, return to the heat, bring to a simmer, reduce the heat to low, and cook until the potato is just tender, about 15 minutes.

Heat the remaining 2 tablespoons oil in a nonstick skillet over medium-high heat. Add the remaining 2 cups shredded cabbage and fry, tossing often, until the cabbage is wilted and nicely browned.

Stir the mustard into the soup, season with salt and pepper to taste, and ladle into serving bowls. Top each serving with a bit of browned shredded cabbage.

Savoy Cabbage Steamed Dumplings with Soy-Miso Dipping Sauce

Making your own dumplings is a bit of a labor of love—it is more time-consuming than most of my recipes, but I do it because I think it's fun and because the dumplings are supertasty. The upside is I can eat as many as I want, because I know they're good for me. MAKES ABOUT 30 DUMPLINGS

For the Dumplings:

2 tablespoons canola oil

1 large leek, halved lengthwise, rinsed well, and very thinly sliced

½ small head of savoy cabbage, cored and very finely shredded

1 medium carrot, finely grated

One 2-inch piece fresh ginger, finely grated

1 fresh Thai chile, thinly sliced

¼ cup dry white wine

1 tablespoon rice wine vinegar

1 tablespoon light soy sauce

About 30 wonton wrappers

For the Dipping Sauce:

3 tablespoons light soy sauce

2 tablespoons rice wine vinegar

1 tablespoon dark brown sugar

2 teaspoons mild miso paste

1 garlic clove, smashed

To make the dumpling filling, heat the oil in a large skillet over medium heat. Add the leek and cook until it begins to soften, about 4 minutes. Add the cabbage, carrot, ginger, and chile and cook, stirring often, until the cabbage has wilted and is starting to soften, about 7 minutes. Add the wine, vinegar, and soy sauce and cook until the mixture is very soft and most of the liquid has cooked off, 7 to 10 minutes longer. Remove from the heat and allow to cool.

To make the dipping sauce, whisk together the soy sauce, vinegar, brown sugar, and miso. Drop in the smashed garlic and set aside.

To make the dumplings, lay a wonton wrapper on a work surface and put a couple teaspoons of the cabbage mixture in the middle. Dip your finger into a little water and wet the edges of the wonton wrapper. Fold over in half and press the edges together to seal, making triangles.

Bring a couple inches of water to a boil in a pot that will snugly hold a bamboo steamer over the top. Grease the surface of one layer of the bamboo steamer with a little canola oil and set as many dumplings in the steamer as will fit without overlapping. Cook the dumplings in batches only 1 layer thick. Cover the steamer and place over the boiling water. Steam until the wonton wrappers turn translucent, about 7 minutes. Remove the garlic from the dipping sauce and serve alongside the dumplings.

Baked Kale and Mushroom Ragout with Parmesan Bread Crumbs

Even though this dish is primarily greens, it is so hearty it could serve as a meal unto itself. Adding a little browned bacon to this otherwise fat-free recipe imparts an incredible amount of flavor, but if you want to make the dish even lighter, or simply vegetarian, just use vegetable stock and leave out the bacon. SERVES 8

I quart chicken, beef, or vegetable stock

2 cups tomato puree

I teaspoon dried thyme

I teaspoon salt

I teaspoon sugar

2 pounds kale, stems removed, leaves roughly chopped

6 large garlic cloves, thinly sliced

10 ounces cremini mushrooms, stems removed and caps thinly sliced

8 ounces bacon (optional), roughly chopped

6 ounces rustic baguette, roughly chopped

4 ounces Parmesan cheese, finely grated (about I cup)

3 tablespoons olive oil

Preheat the oven to 350°F.

Combine the stock, 2 cups of water, tomato puree, thyme, salt, and sugar in a large, tall stockpot. Bring to a simmer over medium-high heat. Add the kale and cook, uncovered, until very tender, about 30 minutes. Use tongs to remove the kale from the simmering liquid, shaking off as much excess liquid as possible, and set it in a 9 × 13-inch baking dish, preferably earthenware. Return the cooking liquid to a simmer, add the garlic and mushrooms, and continue cooking until the mixture has reduced by about half to a thick, saucy consistency, about 30 minutes longer.

Cook the bacon in a large skillet over medium-high heat until it is well browned and nearly all of its fat has rendered, about 10 minutes. Remove the browned bacon bits, leaving the rendered fat behind, and add them to the cooked kale.

Put the chopped baguette into a food processor and grind into fine bread crumbs. Transfer the bread crumbs to a foil-lined baking sheet and toast, shaking once, until very lightly browned, about 10 minutes. Transfer the toasted bread crumbs to a mixing bowl and combine with the Parmesan and olive oil.

Pour the reduced mushroom sauce over the kale and bacon and spread evenly in the baking dish. Spread the bread crumb mixture over the top of the kale, bacon, and mushroom sauce mixture and bake in the oven until the bread crumbs are nicely browned and the sauce starts to bubble up the sides of the baking dish, about 20 minutes.

Spicy Roasted Brussels Sprouts and Butternut Squash

This is a perfect side dish to serve in the fall and winter months. It also makes a healthy holiday accompaniment for roasted meats like the Thanksgiving turkey or the Christmas ham. SERVES 6

1 pound butternut squash flesh, cut into ¾-inch cubes (about 2 cups)

8 ounces Brussels sprouts, bottoms trimmed, halved lengthwise

¼ cup olive oil

Couple dashes of cayenne

5 fresh rosemary sprigs

5 garlic cloves, smashed

Salt and freshly ground black pepper

Preheat the oven to 375°F.

Toss the butternut squash, Brussels sprouts, olive oil, cayenne, rosemary, and garlic together on a large foil-lined baking sheet. Season generously with salt and pepper and cover loosely with a sheet of foil. Bake for 15 to 20 minutes, until the squash and Brussels sprouts are tender. Season again with salt and pepper to taste and spoon into a serving bowl.

Italian Sausage and Savoy Cabbage Linguine

This is a rustic, Northern Italian–inspired pasta dish fit for a cold evening. The sausage is used here more as a flavor accent than as the main event, which cuts down on your overall meat consumption tremendously. SERVES 4 TO 6

---

3 tablespoons olive oil

I pound sweet Italian sausage, casings removed and meat roughly chopped

I teaspoon fennel seeds

½ teaspoon hot red pepper flakes

½ teaspoon dried marjoram

½ head of savoy cabbage, cored and coarsely shredded

¾ cup chicken stock

I pint grape tomatoes

Salt and freshly ground black pepper

I pound linguine

½ cup freshly grated Parmesan cheese

Bring a large pot of water to a boil. Meanwhile, heat the olive oil in a large skillet over medium-high heat. Add the sausage and brown well, using a spoon to break up the meat as you stir. Reduce the heat to medium and stir in the fennel seeds, hot red pepper, marjoram, cabbage, and stock. Cook, partially covered, until the cabbage is tender, about 15 minutes. Add the tomatoes and cook, partially covered, until the tomatoes burst and soften, about 10 minutes longer.

Salt the boiling water, add the linguine, and cook al dente. Drain, reserving ¾ cup of the pasta water, and return the cooked linguine to the pot. Toss with the hot sauce and the pasta water. Season with salt and pepper to taste. To serve, portion into bowls and top with the Parmesan.

Green Curry with Broccoli, Tofu, and Shrimp

There's no cabbage in the title, but broccoli is actually part of the cabbage family. Serve this with brown rice for a delicious and filling meal.

SERVES 6

---

3 tablespoons canola oil

1 medium onion, finely chopped

1 large green bell pepper, cut into thin strips

⅓ cup green curry paste

1 large fresh Thai chile, thinly sliced

One 14-ounce can light coconut milk

2 cups chicken or vegetable stock

2 tablespoons sugar

One 8-ounce can bamboo shoots, drained

One 15-ounce can baby corn, drained

2 cups broccoli florets

1 garlic clove, minced

Juice of ½ lime

7 ounces (½ package) extra-firm tofu, drained and sliced into ¾-inch cubes

8 ounces medium shrimp, peeled and deveined

Heat the oil in a large skillet over medium-high heat. Add the onion and bell pepper and cook, stirring often, until the onion softens and turns nearly translucent, about 7 minutes. Stir in the curry paste and cook until fragrant and steaming, about 3 minutes. Add the chile, coconut milk, stock, sugar, bamboo shoots, and baby corn. Bring to a simmer and cook, partially covered, for 15 minutes.

Put the broccoli florets in a microwave-safe bowl and cover with a plate or bowl. Microwave on high for 2 minutes.

Stir the garlic and lime juice into the curry and add the parcooked broccoli along with the tofu and shrimp. Cook just until the shrimp are cooked through, about 5 minutes.

cabbage vs. broccoli

Broccoli may not look anything at all like a head of cabbage, but the two vegetables are closely related. Their taxonomy is almost identical. Broccoli is known as *Brassica oleracea*, as is cabbage. The only difference is their cultivar group. Cabbage is in the 'Capitata' group; broccoli is in the 'Italica' group.

The two are essentially cousins. And since broccoli is reputed to have all sorts of health benefits, there was no way we could leave it out.

Like cabbage, broccoli contains phytonutrients like sulforaphanes and indole-3-carbinol, which studies have linked to a lower risk of a raft of cancers, from colon to bladder and ovarian, among others. If that weren't enough, a massive study of 100,000 people found that those who regularly consumed broccoli cut their risk of heart disease by about 20 percent.

When you look at its nutrient profile, this should come as no surprise. A single cup of broccoli has a whopping 200 percent of your recommended daily value of vitamin C and 200 percent of the daily value for vitamin K, which helps protect your cells from oxidative damage.

Add it to the right dish, and even a notorious broccoli hater like former president George H. W. Bush might appreciate it. Try it in this curry, and odds are you'll want to have it again and again.

Beef- and Rice-Stuffed
Savoy Cabbage

This is a healthier, more rustic take on the classic Eastern European stuffed cabbage dish, which I absolutely adore. The leaves of savoy cabbage are thin and tender, creating a delicate veil around the beef and rice mixture. SERVES 6 TO 8

I large head of savoy cabbage

2 pounds ground beef

2 eggs

3 garlic cloves, minced

I tablespoon sweet paprika

Few dashes of cayenne

I teaspoon dried thyme

½ teaspoon ground cloves

I tablespoon salt

I teaspoon freshly ground black pepper

I½ cups cooked white rice

One 6-ounce can tomato paste

3 tablespoons ketchup

2 cups beef or chicken stock

Preheat the oven to 350°F.

Bring a large pot of salted water to a simmer. Core the cabbage from the bottom, leaving the head intact. Drop the head of cabbage into the water and use tongs to remove about 14 of the largest leaves of the cabbage as they pull away from the head of cabbage and become tender. Set them aside on a large plate to cool, transfer the pared-down head of cabbage to a cutting board, finely chop it once it has cooled sufficiently to handle, and reserve.

In a large mixing bowl, combine the beef, eggs, garlic, paprika, cayenne, thyme, cloves, salt, pepper, and rice and stir until all the ingredients are well incorporated.

Place about ¼ cup of the meat mixture in the center of each of the whole tender cabbage leaves and wrap up snugly by folding in the sides, folding up the bottom, and tucking under the top. Place the stuffed cabbage leaves in a 9 × 13-inch Pyrex baking dish.

In a large mixing bowl, whisk together the tomato paste, ketchup, stock, and reserved finely chopped cabbage. Pour over the top of the stuffed cabbage leaves. Cover loosely with aluminum foil and bake for 1 hour.

RED WINE

Hands down, the best way to enjoy a bottle of red wine and get most of it into your system is to drink it straight up. But it also has many wonderful applications in the kitchen.

First rule of thumb: Don't cook with your best bottles of wine—drink those. Instead choose wines that are dry, pleasant, and balanced but no great shakes. Whether it's the heating or the combination with other flavors, many of the nuances of a good wine would be lost in the cooking process, so a good cooking wine should be absolutely drinkable but also absolutely average.

OK, so now that that is out of the way, I can get to all the fun ways you can use red wine in your cooking. The French are masters at this. They are so fond of using red wine in their cooking that one of their most classic dishes—coq au vin—is nothing more than chicken soaked in red wine and aromatics and then cooked in it. And it's delicious!

Of course there are more subtle ways of incorporating wine into your cooking. One of the simplest ways is to deglaze a roasting pan after cooking chicken or meat in it to create a wonderfully flavorful sauce in no time. All you have to do is add a couple glugs of red wine, put the roasting pan on top of a large burner or back in the oven, and just wait for it to reduce into a quick pan sauce.

I love using red wine as part of braising liquids. There doesn't seem to be one kind of meat that doesn't succumb to red wine's sly, delicious workings over the course of a long slow braise and turn out tastier for it. Combine stock, red wine, and aromatics and—voilà!—you have the makings of a four-star braise.

Red wine preparations can also go smashingly with more robust fish, like the salmon in my salmon and blackberry recipe (see page 230), and even in all kinds of desserts. One of my favorite and simplest is stone fruit (such as pears, nectarines, and plums) poached in sweetened red wine and served with vanilla and honey Greek yogurt or vanilla ice cream.

These recipes are all sweet and delicious—but not nearly as sweet as all the evidence from epidemiological studies over the years showing that regular (and moderate) consumption of wines can lower the risk of heart disease. This is due at least in part to the widely reported effects of resveratrol, but it may also be a result of tannins, the compounds in red wines that give them their tartness. Studies suggest that tannins, like resveratrol, are good for vascular health.

Braised Lamb, Green Cabbage, and Butter Beans

After an hour and a half in the oven, the cabbage in this recipe nearly melts together with the lamb and the butter beans, creating a rich, succulent one-pot meal. SERVES 4

---

4 lamb shoulder chops

3 tablespoons olive oil

Salt and freshly ground black pepper

1 large onion, finely chopped

2 large carrots, sliced about ⅛ inch thick

½ head of green cabbage (about 1 pound), cored and cut roughly into 1-inch chunks

2 or 3 fresh rosemary sprigs, broken into a few pieces

4 garlic cloves, finely chopped

2 cups chicken, veal, or beef stock

⅔ cup red wine

20 prunes

Two 15-ounce cans butter beans, drained and rinsed

Preheat the oven to 350°F.

Season the lamb chops generously on both sides with salt and pepper.

Heat the olive oil in a large, heavy-bottomed pot over high heat. Brown the lamb chops well on both sides and then set them aside on a large plate. Reduce the heat to medium. Add the onion and carrots and cook, stirring frequently, until the onion is soft and beginning to turn translucent, about 10 minutes.

Return the lamb to the pot and add the cabbage, rosemary, garlic, stock, red wine, prunes, and butter beans. Bring the mixture to a simmer and then transfer it to the oven and cook, uncovered, until the meat is fork-tender and the cooking juices are rich, about 1½ hours.

Serve each chop with a couple ladles of the vegetables and cooking liquid.

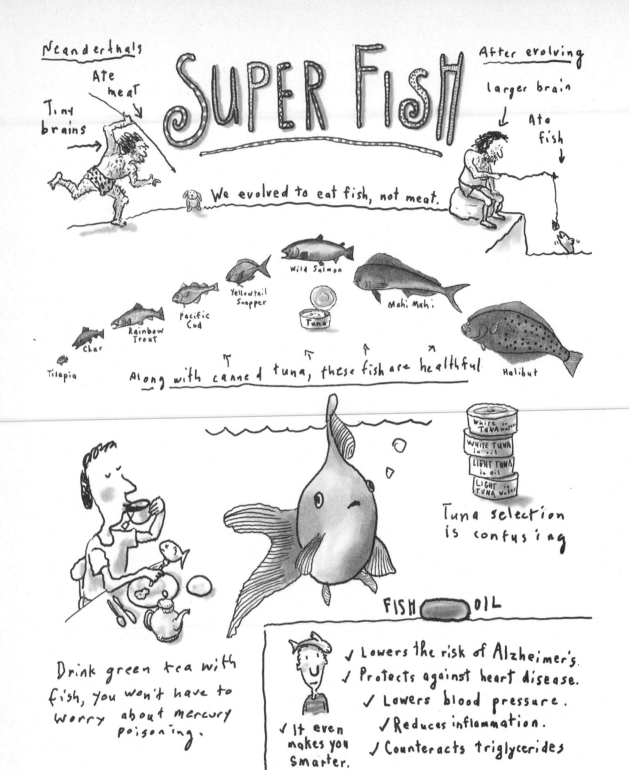

8

SUPER FISH

If you're looking for the Holy Grail of health food, your search may be over.

To understand why, we have to go back hundreds of thousands of years to the prehistoric dinner table—back to the foods that we evolved to eat. Most of us think of our prehistoric ancestors as big-game hunters who chased their red-meat dinners across the African savanna, clubs and spears in hand. It was this strategic ritual that catapulted us to the top of the food chain, forcing us to improvise with tools and rewarding us with the meat and nutrients needed to progress toward modern civilization. That's what we've long been led to believe. But giving all the credit to red meat overlooks what may have been an even more critical ingredient in the story of our evolutionary success.

That's because at some point in our early history the human brain, in a flash of time, underwent a massive and very rapid expansion. Our brains tripled in size from a mere one pound to three, from a mere abacus to a master computer. Our brains grew so huge that mothers were forced to give birth earlier just to accommodate their brainier babies. It was either that or they grow wider birth canals. But that would have limited their ability to run—not the kind of handicap you want when you're trying to stay a step ahead of predators and fierce rivals.

It was with this explosion in brain size that modern man realized his destiny, lifting us out of caves and setting us on the path toward modern civilization while our rivals, the Neanderthals, slowly died out. So what made the difference for early humans?

Some scientists say this all occurred as we began our first culinary forays into the sea.

In recent years, archaeologists have dug up fragments of hooks and nets along the coast of California that were used to catch fish some ten thousand years ago, long before the Pilgrims carved up their first Thanksgiving turkey. In western France, the remains of fish that were shared among different families who hunted together have turned up at campsites as old as forty thousand years. And in caves and sites along the coast of East Africa, scientists have uncovered modern human fossils dating back even further—in some cases more than a hundred thousand years—that lay surrounded by the remains of shellfish and the chewed bones of catfish.

So why was seafood so important to our Paleolithic brethren? Looking at what it has to offer, the reasons become obvious. Seafood contains some of the most powerful brain-nourishing compounds known to man. One of them, DHA, an omega-3 fatty acid, makes up almost half of the essential fatty acids in the human brain. Which is why people with DHA deficiencies suffer cognitive deterioration and other neurological problems.

Don't get us wrong. No one is saying that loading up on fish will leave you needing a larger hat size. But eating fish does seem to help the brain run as smoothly as our owner's manual intended. Plenty of studies show that eating fish at least once a week keeps your mind sharp, lowering the risk of Alzheimer's disease and slowing the decline of mental faculties as you age.

Fish is also at the root of several mysteries that baffled epidemiologists for years. Why is it, for instance, that Inuit populations in the Arctic eat enormous amounts of fat yet suffer little or no coronary heart disease? And how is it that in coastal areas of

Japan, where heavy salt intake consistently drives up rates of hypertension, deaths from heart attacks are rare?

The answer: fish oil. Fatty fish that swim in cold seas comprise a large portion of the diets in the aforementioned populations, and studies show that fish fat lowers blood pressure, blocks compounds that cause inflammation, and prevents cardiovascular damage wrought by triglycerides.

Europeans know this too, which is why in 2004 regulators in almost all European countries approved prescription fish oil for use in heart patients. In countries like France and Italy, where the heart-healthy Mediterranean diet reigns supreme, cardiologists say that sending a heart patient home without a prescription for fish oil would almost be considered malpractice.

So explains my turnaround, from a lifelong vegan who followed his parents' ways to a *New York Times* health reporter and unabashed fishmonger. But lucky for us, what's good for the heart and good for the brain is even better for the palate.

Dave and I are sometimes known to butt heads on some of our creations. But when I busted out the science on fish oil, there was no dispute. For Dave, as a chef, the thought of cooking with a food laden with fat that's rich *and* superhealthy was too good to let go.

It's simple. Fat makes food taste good. Scientists even believe we have taste receptors on our tongues that are specifically for fat—put there, for evolutionary purposes, to ensure that we ate high-energy meals back in the days when food was hard to come by (this, of course, was way before we invented trans fats and the deep fryer).

For a chef, fat is king. Get Dave going on the finer points of cooking seafood and he waxes on and on about properly prepared fish flesh, throwing out words that most men would use only to describe *other* carnal pleasures. Words like *silky, succulent,* and *buttery.*

"Dude, take it down a notch," I once had to tell him.

Switching gears, he talks about the "versatility" of fish, a trait you can chalk up to "their sweet, mild flesh that's like a clean canvas ready for strokes of color." As any true fish lover, including Dave, will tell you, sometimes the best thing to do with a great piece of fish, quite simply, is to rub it with olive oil, salt, and pepper and stick it under a hot broiler. But that wouldn't make for much of a cookbook, so Dave has come up with a bunch of really delicious yet simple recipes that incorporate the varieties of fish that are hands down the best for you to eat.

Picking some varieties over others, however, forces us to consider the sad fact that our fish story is not entirely a love affair. Our Paleolithic ancestors plucked their meals from oceans that were clean and vibrant, whereas nowadays our seafood comes from seas and lakes that increasingly are on life support, thanks to problems with pollution that are nearly all manmade.

What we spew from our smokestacks, exhaust pipes, and industrial farms finds its way into the food chain. And ultimately, onto our dinner plates. Isn't karma cruel?

But don't despair. In the following pages, we show you how to maximize the nutritional benefits of fish while minimizing your exposure to the stuff you *don't* want. We've done the research and pored through the studies, and we've carefully selected the tastiest, most beneficial fish. Now we'll show you how to cook them in ways that send those fat-loving taste receptors into overdrive.

So no more excuses. It's time to step it up with fish fat!

Tuna with Chickpeas, Tomatoes, Baby Arugula, and Fresh Oregano

This is one of my all-time favorite lunch dishes. It is satisfying and flavorful while being fresh and healthy. Plus it's superquick and simple to make, a key point when it comes to preparing lunch or dinner in a hurry.

SERVES 4

Two 10-ounce cans olive oil–packed light tuna

One 15-ounce can chickpeas, drained and rinsed

Juice of 1 lemon

6 ounces cherry or grape tomatoes, quartered

¼ cup olive oil

1 large shallot, minced

3 or 4 large leaves from fresh oregano sprigs, to taste

About 2 ounces baby arugula (preferably wild)

Salt and freshly ground black pepper

Combine the tuna, chickpeas, lemon juice, tomatoes, olive oil, shallots, oregano, and arugula in a large mixing bowl. Toss well and then season with salt and pepper to taste.

canned tuna

Open any pantry in America, and you're likely to find a can of tuna—Americans eat about a billion pounds of the stuff every year. Despite its role as a kitchen staple, many people couldn't tell you the difference between all those cans that line your local supermarket shelves.

Canned tuna comes packed in several ways. There's solid and chunk. Solid is one piece of tuna loin cut to fit the can, while "chunk" is exactly what it sounds like—chunks of tuna, rather than one solid piece. Tuna also comes canned in different liquids, either water or various types of oil, including olive. We find olive oil–packed tuna by far the most flavorful option, and the olive oil is much healthier than the other oil choices.

But the most important differentiator when it comes to canned tuna is the kind of tuna that's actually in the can. There are literally dozens of species of fish that are considered tuna: albacore, bigeye, bluefin, and yellowfin among them.

So-called white tuna can contain only albacore tuna. This is considered a premium grade of canned tuna, but the problem is that albacore's size and high position on the food chain mean its flesh contains higher amounts of mercury and other heavy metals.

It's for this reason that we don't recommend albacore canned tuna, but rather "light" tuna, which primarily uses skipjack, a smaller species of tuna with very low levels of mercury. It's also mild and pleasant in flavor, making it a go-to fish option.

One small caveat, though: Regulations allow for cans of "light" tuna to contain a small percentage of other kinds of tuna, mostly just to fill out the can. This means there's a small chance that some tuna with slightly higher levels of mercury might find its way into your can. But the figure is low, at around 5 percent.

For all the healthy benefits (and eating pleasure!) that you'll get out of "light" tuna, it's a small risk to live with.

Smoked Salmon Plate

Smoked salmon is one of my favorite foods, and I've eaten a lot of it over the years, so it comes as a relief that it is also good for you. Serve it with some toasted dark bread or any other whole wheat or whole-grain breads or bagels and you'll be in heaven. SERVES 4

8 ounces smoked salmon, thinly sliced

About ¼ cup thick Greek-style yogurt

Freshly ground black pepper

2 shallots, halved lengthwise and thinly sliced crosswise

3 tablespoons drained capers

Olive oil to taste

Juice of 1 lemon

About 2 tablespoons fresh dill leaves, roughly chopped

Divide the salmon among 4 plates, laying the pieces around the center of the plate. Place a good dollop of yogurt in the middle of each plate. Lightly season the salmon and the yogurt with black pepper; then scatter the sliced shallots and capers over it all. Drizzle each plate with the olive oil and a squeeze of lemon juice and finally garnish with the chopped dill.

mercury be gone!

Stick with the fish listed in these pages and you'll maximize your intake of omega-3s while minimizing your exposure to mercury. But you can take additional steps to reduce your exposure even further.

For starters, the next time you cut into a piece of fish, pour yourself a cup of green tea.

Food scientists at Purdue University found that drinking tea could prevent contaminants in seafood from entering your system. The researchers showed that when mackerel was combined with tea extract, the levels of mercury that were subsequently absorbed plummeted by more than 90 percent.

Certain compounds in green tea, particularly one class of compounds called *catechins*, bind to the toxins and sweep them out of your system. Scientists believe that may be the reason some communities along the St. Lawrence River just east of Montreal and the Bay of Fundy in Nova Scotia—populations that eat loads of fish and drink lots of tea—have mysteriously low levels of mercury in their systems.

A similar pattern has emerged in the Brazilian Amazon, where pockets of people who subsist largely on fish have been shown to have surprisingly low levels of mercury. Except in this case it appears that it's tropical fruit doing the trick. When people who ate equal amounts of fish were compared, those who ate fruit more frequently had *significantly* less mercury in their systems. They absorbed about a third of the amount from the same quantities of fish, apparently because of antagonistic nutrients in fruit that help eliminate toxins from the system. It's a phenomenon that's been documented in a number of studies since it was first observed in 2003.

More tea, more fruit. Eating fish just keeps getting better and better . . .

Halibut, Braised Fennel, Cauliflower, and Cherry Tomatoes over Penne

Halibut is a very tender, succulent fish, and braised fennel has the same qualities, so the textures work nicely together. The penne makes this dish a one-plate meal; use whole wheat penne if you have it. SERVES 4

½ cup olive oil

1 fennel bulb, cored and thinly sliced lengthwise

1 large onion, halved lengthwise and thinly sliced

½ head of cauliflower, cored and broken into small florets

1 teaspoon hot red pepper flakes

½ cup dry white wine

12 ounces cherry tomatoes

Salt and freshly ground black pepper

1 pound halibut, cut into roughly 1-inch chunks

Leaves from 1 small bunch of fresh basil

Heat a heavy-bottomed pot or Dutch oven over medium heat. Add the olive oil, fennel, onion, cauliflower, and hot red pepper. Cook with the pot partially covered, stirring from time to time, until the fennel and onion have "melted," about 15 minutes.

Add the wine and tomatoes and cover the pot. Cook until the tomatoes have burst open and started to render their juice, about 10 minutes longer. Season the mixture with salt and pepper to taste.

Reduce the heat to medium-low; slide in the fish. Cover the pot and cook about 5 minutes longer, just until the fish is cooked through but still tender and flaky.

Remove the dish from the heat, stir in the basil leaves, and season with salt and pepper to taste one more time before serving.

the new surf 'n' turf

Forget steak and lobster. This is the new surf 'n' turf.

This unusual pairing of halibut and cauliflower blows me away every time. Combined, they taste amazing, and as a tag team they synergize and multiply each other's most healthful benefits.

Cauliflower contains sulforaphane (as does broccoli, page 161, and the other cruciferous vegetables you read about in the cabbage chapter). You should have it in your diet because it's a powerful cancer-fighting compound. And biochemists have found in studies that it does its job about ten times better when it's combined with selenium, a mineral with antioxidant properties. Put them together and they're more than just the sum of their parts.

That's where the halibut comes in: it's loaded with selenium. Combining it with cauliflower or the other cruciferous veggies creates a meal that packs a power punch. You can find selenium in many other types of fish, particularly tuna and cod. That's one reason we've united tuna and arugula in an awesome salad. The message here is: always combine your fish with veggies. Besides, it'll make Mom proud.

Poached Arctic Char

Arctic char fillet looks a lot like salmon fillet, but it's less fatty and milder in flavor. That's why it requires a cooking method, like poaching, that is very gentle. SERVES 4

6 cups fish or seafood stock, preferably homemade

4 or 5 fresh thyme sprigs, plus fresh thyme leaves for garnish

3 bay leaves

Salt and freshly ground black pepper

About 1¼ pounds arctic char fillet, skinned and cut into 4 equal portions

8 ounces green beans, preferably *haricots verts*

8 ounces red potatoes, steamed or boiled until tender and quartered

2 shallots, minced (about ½ cup)

2 tablespoons whole-grain mustard

¼ cup thick Greek-style yogurt

¼ cup sour cream

Juice of 1 lemon

Bring the fish stock, thyme sprigs, and bay leaves to a simmer in a large pot or fish poacher. Season with salt and pepper to taste and let the stock simmer for 10 minutes. Reduce the heat so that the stock is barely simmering and slide in the pieces of fish. Cook for about 7 minutes, just until the fish is cooked through but still holds its shape. Remove the fish and set aside. Reserve the hot stock.

Meanwhile, steam the green beans until bright green, just a few minutes, and throw in the potato pieces at the tail end of the cooking to reheat them thoroughly. Remove the green beans and potatoes from the heat.

Whisk together the shallots, mustard, yogurt, sour cream, lemon juice, and ⅓ cup of the reserved stock. Toss with the hot beans and potatoes. Season with salt and pepper.

Divide the warm salad among 4 shallow bowls. Place a piece of fish on top of each and garnish with some fresh thyme leaves.

brain food

Need any more evidence that fish is brain food?

You can find it by looking at the impact that eating fish has on infant development. Mothers who eat more fish give birth to children who have better motor and cognitive development.

One study of 25,000 small children by researchers at Harvard, for example, found that those whose mothers had been eating moderate amounts of fish while pregnant and nursing—mostly the very-low-mercury types of fish like cod, salmon, and mackerel—were 25 percent more likely to have higher development scores than other children at six months and almost 30 percent more likely to have higher scores at eighteen months. The women ate about 12 ounces of fish a week, the rough equivalent of two or three servings.

Incidentally, that is exactly the amount of fish that health authorities have long said pregnant women and nursing mothers can safely consume. And we know from other studies that early exposure to omega-3s—which are also found in breast milk—can result in higher IQ scores as well.

Of course, if you're pregnant or nursing, you should also be wary of potential exposure to contaminants. But you can lower the risk by following the Food and Drug Administration's recommendations. Limit yourself to two meals of fish a week and always avoid eating shark, swordfish, king mackerel, and tilefish, which contain the highest levels of mercury. Salmon and canned light tuna are great alternatives.

Almond and Herb Baked Tilapia

Tilapia has quickly become one of the most affordable and widely available fish at the supermarket. It has sweet, mild, meaty flesh that is tender as long as you don't overcook it. This almond and herb topping is vibrant and flavorful, and the toasted sliced almonds add some nice crunch. But the topping also serves double duty, locking in the moisture of the fish. Lots of good extra virgin olive oil helps the cause too! SERVES 4

⅓ cup olive oil, plus more for drizzling

Juice and grated zest of 1 lemon

1 cup sliced raw almonds

2 garlic cloves, minced or pressed

¼ cup very finely chopped fresh parsley leaves

Salt and freshly ground black pepper

4 large, thick tilapia fillets (about 6 to 8 ounces each)

Preheat the oven to 400°F.

Toss the olive oil, lemon juice and zest, almonds, garlic, and parsley together in a mixing bowl and season with salt and pepper to taste.

Place the pieces of tilapia on a large baking sheet lined with aluminum foil. Season lightly with salt and pepper and drizzle lightly with olive oil.

Divide the almond and herb mixture among the four pieces of fish and smooth the mixture over each piece to create an even coating.

Bake until the almond mixture has browned slightly and the fish is cooked through and flakes easily, about 15 minutes.

farmed vs. wild fish

By now most people know that wild salmon—the third most popular seafood in America, behind shrimp and tuna—is healthier than farmed salmon. But is wild fish always better than farmed?

Well, not exactly.

Fish caught in the wild are plucked from the ocean by fishermen using nets and traps, while species raised on farms are kept in pens and cages, much like more traditional commercial livestock. For larger, carnivorous species like salmon, life on a farm can be harsh. They're kept in close quarters, which increases the risk of infections like sea lice, and fed a heavy diet of other fish that may contain contaminants.

Other farmed fish may vary in quality, depending on their country of origin. Farmed tilapia, for example, are generally low in contaminants, except when they come from farms in China and Taiwan, where pollution and lax management lead to poor-quality fish that you *don't* want on your plate.

The same goes for shellfish like mussels and shrimp. They're generally better when raised on farms because they're kept on healthy plant-food diets. But shrimp imported from China should be avoided. The quality is so poor, and the potential levels of chemicals so risky, that the Food and Drug Administration imposed a ban in 2007 on all shrimp imported from China (along with Chinese imports of catfish, basa, dace, and eel).

Figuring out what's good for you and good for the environment is no easy task. But rest easy. We did some research, crunched some numbers, and pored through mounds of data to come up with a list of the healthiest, tastiest fish available—fish you'll find pretty much anywhere. Here's how they size up:

Fish	Environmentally Friendly?	Omega-3s	Mercury and Other Contaminants
Pacific Halibut	Yes	High	Low
Tilapia (U.S.)	Yes	Good	Low
Wild Salmon	Yes	Extremely High	Low
Rainbow Trout	Yes	Very High	Low
Mahimahi (U.S.)	Good	Good	Low
Pacific Cod (No Atlantic/No Black)	Yes	Good	Low
Canned Light Tuna	Yes	Good	Low to moderate (because some cans may occasionally contain yellowfin, which has more mercury than skipjack)
Yellowtail Snapper	Yes	Good	Low to Moderate
Farmed Arctic Char	Yes	High	Low

Based on analyses conducted by the Food and Drug Administration, the Environmental Defense Fund, and the Monterey Bay Aquarium Seafood Watch program.

Lemongrass, Lime, and Snapper Soup

Whenever I'm feeling under the weather, I find myself craving this soup. It is fragrant, light, and spicy, and the fresh snapper satisfies. I always leave the skin of the snapper on the fillet, because it is thin and delicate and keeps the fish intact while it cooks. Whatever you do, don't cook the fish longer than just a few minutes, as the fish is so tender it can easily get overcooked. That also means you need to serve the soup as soon as it is ready. SERVES 6

1 fresh lemongrass stalk, cut into 1-inch pieces

1 tablespoon finely grated fresh ginger

2 small fresh red Thai chiles, thinly sliced

2 large shallots, peeled and very thinly sliced

1 cup cored and chopped tomato

1 quart fish or seafood stock, preferably homemade

1 cup light coconut milk

Salt and freshly ground black pepper

About 1½ pounds skin-on snapper fillet, cut into about 1-inch pieces

Juice and grated zest of 1 small lime

1 small bunch of fresh cilantro, tough stems removed, roughly chopped

Combine the lemongrass, ginger, chiles, shallots, tomato, stock, and coconut milk in a large pot and bring the mixture to a simmer over medium heat. Cook for about 20 minutes. Remove the pieces of lemongrass. Season the broth with salt and pepper to taste.

Reduce the heat to medium-low and slide the fish pieces into the broth along with the lime juice and zest. Cook for about 5 minutes, until the fish has just cooked through.

Divide the soup among 6 bowls and garnish each with chopped fresh cilantro.

Rainbow Trout Baked with Red Onions, Lemon, and Rosemary

Even though it is probably the easiest of preparations, serving a whole fish is very special. And because you leave the flesh entirely intact, it retains all of its natural moisture and flavor. When it comes to cooking fish whole, I always prefer the simplest of preparations, as you can tell from this recipe. SERVES 4

---

1 whole farmed rainbow trout (about 2 pounds), gutted and cleaned

Salt and freshly ground black pepper

Olive oil

1 lemon, halved lengthwise and thinly sliced crosswise

A few fresh rosemary sprigs

1 small red onion, halved lengthwise and thinly sliced crosswise

Preheat the oven to 375°F.

Place the trout on a baking sheet lined with aluminum foil and season inside and out with salt and pepper. Rub generously all over with olive oil.

Stuff the cavity of the fish with as much lemon, rosemary, and red onion as will fit and place whatever remains over the top and around the fish.

Drizzle generously with more olive oil and bake for about 25 minutes, until the fish flakes easily away from the bone and the red onions have started to take on some color.

Fillet the fish at the table and serve with the cooked red onions, lemon, plus the starch of your choice.

Rosemary-Grilled Mahimahi with Red Pepper and Radicchio Relish

Mahimahi is a meaty, potentially tough fish, so a quick grilling is the perfect way to cook it. Instead of heavily seasoning the fish, I prefer to serve it with something very flavorful. I take advantage of having a hot grill or grill pan already in use to cook down some radicchio while the fish is finishing up. I then toss it with roasted red peppers, briny green olives, sun-dried tomatoes, and a bit of balsamic vinegar. SERVES 4

About 1¼ pounds mahimahi fillet, skin removed and cut into 4 equal portions

¼ cup olive oil, plus more for the peppers and for drizzling

2 large fresh rosemary sprigs, torn in half

Juice of 1 lemon

Salt and freshly ground black pepper

2 red bell peppers

1 medium head of radicchio, cored and cut lengthwise into eighths

⅓ cup pitted green olives, roughly chopped

¼ cup sun-dried tomatoes packed in olive oil, finely chopped

3 tablespoons balsamic vinegar

Preheat the broiler to the highest heat and position a rack about 8 inches from the heat element.

Marinate the mahimahi by putting the fish pieces in a large resealable plastic bag along with ¼ cup of olive oil, the rosemary, and the lemon juice. Season lightly with salt and pepper. Seal the bag, massage the ingredients together, and set aside.

Rub the peppers with olive oil, season generously with salt, and place on a baking sheet lined with aluminum foil. Broil the peppers, turning every so often, until all the sides have been well blackened, about 30 minutes. Transfer the peppers to a mixing bowl and cover tightly with plastic wrap. Let sit until the peppers have cooled and completely collapsed, about 20 minutes. Peel and discard the blackened skin, remove the stems and seeds, and roughly chop the pepper flesh.

Heat a grill pan over high heat for about 7 minutes. Grill the fish for about 4 minutes per side, leaving room for the radicchio. As soon as you have turned the fish over, sprinkle the radicchio with some salt, drizzle with some olive oil, and cook on the grill pan just until wilted and tender. The fish and the radicchio should come off the grill roughly at the same time, but the radicchio may take a bit longer, depending on the size of your grill pan and the amount of heat your stovetop can put out.

Toss the radicchio with the chopped roasted red peppers, olives, sun-dried tomatoes, and balsamic vinegar. Season with salt to taste, if necessary, and serve alongside the grilled fish and a starch of your choice.

Zucchini-Layered Salmon with Stewed Eggplant

The nice thing about salmon is that it can stand up to a range of flavors and preparations. It is delicious almost any way you prepare it, whether it's on the grill, in the oven, or simply panfried. Here I'm pairing the salmon with a riff on ratatouille, but instead of combining the zucchini with the eggplant and tomatoes, I layer very thin slices of zucchini on top of the fish to keep the salmon as moist as possible. It also makes for an impressive presentation. SERVES 6

For the Eggplant:

1 large eggplant, peeled and cut into roughly 1-inch cubes

Kosher salt

½ cup olive oil

1 large yellow onion, halved lengthwise and thinly sliced

½ teaspoon hot red pepper flakes

3 tablespoons red wine vinegar

2 cups chopped canned tomato, with juices

3 large garlic cloves, finely chopped

1 tablespoon sugar

For the Salmon:

About 1⅔ pounds salmon, preferably wild, cut into 6 equal portions

Salt and freshly ground black pepper

Olive oil

1 small zucchini, very thinly sliced with a mandoline

¼ cup dry white wine

Juice of ½ lemon

Preheat the oven to 400°F.

To prepare the eggplant, place it in a large colander in the sink and sprinkle generously with kosher salt. Stir and allow to sit for 15 or 20 minutes to release some of its water.

Heat the olive oil in a large pot over medium-high heat. Pat the eggplant dry with a couple paper towels, add the eggplant to the pot and immediately stir vigorously into the hot oil. Add the onion and hot red pepper and stir them into the eggplant. Reduce the heat to medium, partially cover the pot, and cook for about 15 minutes, stirring every 5 minutes, until the vegetables have softened. Stir in the vinegar, tomato, garlic, and sugar, reduce the heat to medium-low, and cook for 45 minutes longer.

Put the salmon on a baking sheet lined with aluminum foil. Season the fish lightly with salt and pepper and drizzle lightly with olive oil. Toss the thinly sliced zucchini with some more olive oil, salt, and pepper and distribute the slices evenly among the pieces of fish. Smooth the zucchini slices firmly against the fish to form a thin layer on top. Pour the white wine and lemon juice over the top of the fish and bake for about 15 minutes, just until the zucchini starts to brown. Serve the salmon on a bed of the hot stewed eggplant.

marinade magic

If you're a grill lover, the marinade in this dish will awaken your taste buds and knock your socks off, but it's also there for your health.

Lighting up the Weber and grilling piles of crispy meat is an all-American art form, as much a cherished pastime as football and the Fourth of July. But grilling meat, poultry, and fish creates substances that can be hazardous to your health. One of them is a group of compounds called *heterocyclic amines*, and they're created when the amino acids in meat and fish are broken down at high temperatures. The U.S. Department of Health and Human Services lists these compounds as known carcinogens.

No surprise, then, that epidemiological studies by the National Cancer Institute show that people who eat lots of grilled or barbecued meat, particularly when it's well done, have higher rates of some cancers.

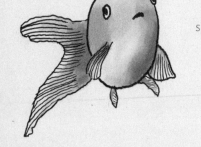

That's where marinating comes to the rescue. It has a strong protective effect. Marinating your fish for even just a few minutes can cut the amount of heterocyclic amines formed by as much as 99 percent. And marinades that contain an acidic base—like citrus juice or vinegar—are best. That's why we're going with olive oil and lemon juice. It's best for your body and pairs deliciously with a slice of succulent mahimahi. Time to warm up the grill.

Broiled Asian-Style Pacific Cod

Cod is loved worldwide for its very mild flavor and light texture. Here I throw a bold, sweet, and spicy Asian-style marinade its way. Cod is overfished in the Atlantic, so please look for Pacific cod. SERVES 4

3 tablespoons soy sauce

½ teaspoon dark sesame oil

3 tablespoons canola oil

3 tablespoons mirin or dry white wine

3 garlic cloves, minced

1 tablespoon dark brown sugar

1 tablespoon grated fresh ginger

4 ounces white mushrooms, thinly sliced

1 large fresh red chile, thinly sliced

1¼ pounds cod fillet, cut into 4 equal portions

8 ounces snap peas, cut on an angle into ¼-inch strips

Combine all the ingredients except the snap peas in a large resealable plastic bag. Close the bag and massage all the ingredients together. Let sit for 30 minutes at room temperature or up to overnight in the refrigerator.

Preheat the broiler to the highest heat and position the oven rack in the middle.

Remove the fish fillets from the bag and brush off the excess marinade. Place the fillets on one half of a medium baking pan lined with aluminum foil. Dump the remaining contents of the bag alongside the fish on the other half of the baking pan. Place under the broiler and cook for 10 to 12 minutes, shaking once or twice. Add the snap peas halfway through the cooking and cook until the fish flakes easily, the mushrooms have browned, and the peas are tender.

Place a piece of fish in the middle of a plate and spoon some sauce, mushrooms, and peas over the top. A side of brown rice is my favorite accompaniment.

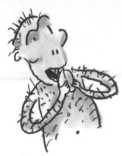

NUTS

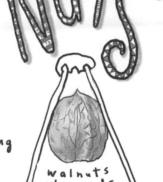

Australopithecus Africanus had strong jaws for opening nuts, the staple of their diet.

walnuts
almonds
peanuts
pecans
cashews
pinenuts
hazelnuts

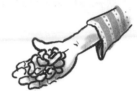

A handful of nuts is all you need.

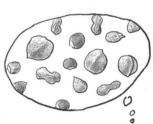

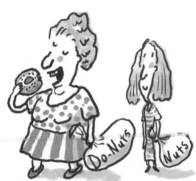

Do-Nuts   Nuts

Walnuts help you sleep.

Eating nuts makes you skinny

And maybe even rich*

*An occasionally true statement.

Nuts Are Healthful, too!

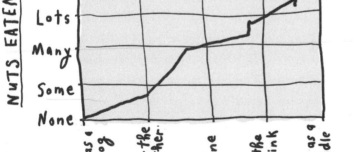

NUTS EATEN

Gobs
Lots
Many
Some
None

Sick as a dog · Under the weather · Fine · In the pink · Fit as a fiddle

HEALTH

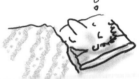

In a nutshell: Nuts are good for you. Eat them.

9

NUTS

When was the last time you ate a handful of walnuts or hazelnuts?

Be completely honest. It probably wasn't anytime in the last couple weeks. Or maybe even in the last year. In fact if you're anything like the average American, it was probably that time you had that bag of trail mix a while back, when there was nothing else to eat. Or perhaps the closest you've come to a hazelnut is that jar of Nutella sitting in your cupboard (sorry, that doesn't count).

But did you know that just a handful of walnuts contains a full day's worth of omega-3 fatty acids? Or that the same amount of almonds contains more protein than an entire egg and no cholesterol at all?

We hate to break the bad news to you and the rest of America, but your ancestors would be disappointed. No, not the ancestors of two generations ago. We mean your ancestors of two million years ago, *Australopithecus africanus,* who literally relied on the nutrients in nuts for their survival.

We know this because millions of years ago our ancestors looked very different than we do today, with jaws and teeth that were exceptionally large and even columns of thick bone running alongside their noses. For a while, scientists assumed that *Australopithecus* needed these juggernaut

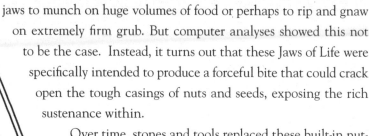

walnuts
almonds
peanuts
pecans
cashews
pinenuts
hazelnuts

jaws to munch on huge volumes of food or perhaps to rip and gnaw on extremely firm grub. But computer analyses showed this not to be the case. Instead, it turns out that these Jaws of Life were specifically intended to produce a forceful bite that could crack open the tough casings of nuts and seeds, exposing the rich sustenance within.

Over time, stones and tools replaced these built-in nut-crackers, allowing the jaws of early man to evolve into the more gentle manifestation that you see today.

But while the shape and contours of the human face may be different, the health powers of nuts like almonds, cashews, hazelnuts, and walnuts haven't changed one bit. Each is a powerhouse of all-natural preventive medicine that just might lengthen your life: protein, fiber, heart-strengthening fats, antioxidants, and a slew of awesome vitamins.

And yet most people ignore these foods as if they were last year's stock tips.

It is not terribly difficult to see why. Nuts are widely misperceived as fattening, unsatisfying, and nutritionally bankrupt—in other words, a throwaway food. But this couldn't be further from reality. Let's call them what they are: food fallacies.

The truth is that a slew of research shows that people who eat nuts are actually more likely to *lose* weight than gain it, and are more likely to report feeling satiated after meals. They also experience more improvements in their energy levels and cardiovascular and cognitive profiles.

There's no doubt nuts are one of the most important foods you can add to your plate. We chose these four varieties—along with peanuts, technically a legume—for two reasons. First, each is hearty and filling, with a rich, buttery mouthfeel, yet each is distinct in flavor. Finding new ways to incorporate them into recipes can be a never-ending exercise. Second, they are quite simply chock-full of great stuff.

You don't have to take it from us.

Take it from the researchers at Loma Linda University who conducted a prominent study in the *British Journal of Nutrition* in 2006 that looked at the diets of thousands of people. They found that people who ate a mere four servings of nuts every week experienced nearly a 40 percent reduction in their risk of coronary heart disease compared with those who rarely or never ate nuts. And better yet, for every additional serving that a person ate beyond those four, there was an additional 8 percent reduction in risk.

As if that weren't enough, another study came along the same year and reported that people who ate just one serving a week of nuts or foods that contain them—like peanut butter—saw an 11 percent drop in their risk of dying from cardiovascular disease. Eating these foods up to four times a week meant a 20 percent decline in risk.

Numbers like that are hard to ignore.

So what's behind their magic?

It's simple. Nuts are loaded with heart-healthy fats, including oleic acid, the kind found in olive oil, and omega-3s, which raise your levels of HDL cholesterol (the good kind) and lower your triglycerides (bad stuff). One small serving of walnuts alone (about ¼ cup) contains 95 percent of the recommended daily value of omega-3 fatty acids. I'll bet you thought they were found only in fish. When you consider that most Americans don't get nearly enough omega-3s, it's clear that a tiny amount could make a huge difference.

And yet even though nuts are loaded with healthful fat, they won't actually *make* you fat. If you're one of the many people who think the opposite, then throw out everything you've heard. It's time for the facts.

When scientists in Spain, for example, followed nearly nine thousand men and women over twenty-eight months for a study of weight gain that was published in the *Journal of Obesity*, they found that people who consumed nuts at least twice a week were 30 percent less likely to pack on pounds than those who never ate them. In fact, people who rarely ate them actually put on far more weight.

As the scientists summed it up, "Frequent nut consumption was associated with a reduced risk of weight gain (5 kilograms or more). These results support the recommendation of nut consumption as an important component of a cardio-protective diet and also allay fears of possible weight gain."

In case you were wondering, 5 kilograms translates to roughly 11 pounds.

Still not convinced?

Keep in mind that other studies have shown that women who added about 350 calories' worth of almonds a day to their diets didn't gain weight, even when they didn't cut back on other calories or step up their levels of exercise. And that women who followed a low-calorie diet with almonds included lost more weight than those who ate the same calories but without almonds.

The reason, in a nutshell (come on, we had to go there), is that nuts make you feel full while also ramping up your body's ability to burn fat. Each is brimming with antioxidants like vitamin E and minerals like magnesium. But each has its own unique blend and proportions.

Of course, to reap the benefits of these foods, you can't simply add them on top of a high-calorie, high-fat Western diet and expect them to work wonders. The key is to eat them in place of those other foods. I've always tried to get my fill by snacking on packets of trail mix that I get from vending machines in the newsroom at the *Times*. But that'll only get you so far.

Thankfully Dave has the culinary chops to bring out their full potential. From a cook's perspective, Dave tells me the three best things going for nuts are their texture, their fat content, and, obviously, their flavor. As he puts it:

I rely on nuts for textural contrast time and again. This is particularly true with salads, where a pile of well-dressed tender greens just cries out for some crunch. But even when it comes to meaty dishes, like the Chinese classic kung pao chicken (page 208), the satisfying crunch from the peanuts truly makes the dish. Sometimes a good nutty flavor is what makes a dish great. The crushed peanuts in my green mango salad (page 197) provide the most dominant flavor. And what would Nutella be without the flavor from hazelnuts—quelle horreur!

But taking advantage of the healthy fat content of nuts is probably the most fun part of this task. You can easily achieve the consistency of heavy cream dishes with nothing more than a handful of raw nuts, as I do with cashews in the garam masala spiced chicken recipe you'll find on page 205. Anahad was so astounded with the creamy richness of this dish that he had a hard time accepting that it contained not a single drop of butter or ghee.

Personally, I've been familiar with the astonishing transformative nature of nuts from an early age because my father used to make his own peanut butter, an occasion that always provided me with entertainment. I loved getting right up close to the food processor, holding my ears, and watching as a big bag of whole peanuts was transformed into a warm, smooth, and creamy mass. Once my father used his fresh peanut butter to make an Africa-inspired soup, and, frankly, while the soup wasn't a great hit (sorry, Dad), I distinctly remember its mouth-coating richness.

But nuts also have the potential for lightness, as you'll discover with my grandmother's recipe for almond lemon sponge cake (page 210). There's no weight or sense of richness that comes from the ground almonds, only their delicate crunch. And when you finely grind nuts, not only is there no heaviness or creamy richness; they actually can substitute for dry flour in many baking recipes! The most classic example of this is a torte. The rich and chocolaty flourless torte at the end of the chapter is a good example of their binding power.

Nuts refuse to be pigeonholed. They refuse to serve just one purpose. With the slightest of manipulations, they change into something drastically different. They're like chameleons of the food world—except that whether they're ground into a thick paste or mixed into a salad, they remain equally good for you.

Slivered Almond and Carrot Salad

The cool freshness of the carrots, the crunch of the almonds, the sweetness of the raisins, the bulk of the kasha, and the zing of the dressing makes each bite interesting. SERVES 6 TO 8

For the Salad:

½ cup golden raisins

¾ cup boiling water

2 tablespoons canola oil

I large red onion, finely chopped

I pound carrots, coarsely grated

1½ cups sliced almonds, lightly toasted

⅓ cup finely chopped flat-leaf parsley

I cup kasha, cooked according to package directions

For the Dressing:

3 tablespoons honey

¼ cup canola oil

¼ cup cider vinegar

2 tablespoons soy sauce

One 2-inch piece fresh ginger, finely grated

Put the raisins in a small mixing bowl and cover with the boiling water. Cover the bowl with plastic wrap and set the raisins aside to soak.

Heat the oil in a small skillet over medium heat and add the onion. Cook, partially covered, stirring frequently, until the onion is soft and sweet, about 7 minutes. Remove from the heat, transfer the cooked onion to a plate, and set aside to cool.

Combine the carrots, almonds, parsley, and kasha in a large mixing bowl. Drain any remaining liquid from the raisins and add them to the carrot mixture along with the cooled onion.

Whisk the dressing ingredients together in a small bowl; then pour the dressing over the top of the carrot mixture and toss well until fully incorporated.

Spicy Green Mango and Peanut Salad

This is a great way to put those underripe mangoes to good use. The salad is a touch tangy, spicy, and salty, which is why the vibrant fresh herbs add so much to the dish. SERVES 6 TO 8

2 large, slightly underripe mangoes (about 1 pound each)

Juice of 2 limes

1 teaspoon Asian fish sauce

1 teaspoon Tabasco sauce

1 large shallot, halved lengthwise and very thinly sliced crosswise

¾ cup unsalted peanuts, pulsed in a food processor until finely chopped

Leaves from 1 bunch of fresh cilantro, roughly chopped

Leaves from 1 bunch of fresh mint, roughly chopped

Use a paring knife to remove the skin from the mangoes and cut the flesh from the pit in large, long chunks; then thinly slice the chunks lengthwise.

Combine the lime juice, fish sauce, and Tabasco sauce in a large mixing bowl. Add the mango, shallot, peanuts, and herbs. Toss gently but thoroughly and serve immediately.

peanut salad

You don't have to look far to find more potential advantages to eating peanuts. They may even slash the risk of colon cancer.

In one study published in 2006, for example, scientists followed more than 20,000 men and women, looking at the different foods they consumed and whether they were linked to this deadly disease, one of the most common cancers in the world. They found that eating just two or more servings of peanuts a week lowered the risk of the disease by nearly 60 percent in women and almost 30 percent in men.

It's not clear why they might have this effect (perhaps because of their high fiber content), and eating more peanuts is certainly no guarantee. But the potential for added protection is nice to think about while munching on this peanut-heavy salad.

walnuts
almonds
peanuts
pecans
cashews
pine nuts
hazelnuts

Spiced Rosemary Cashews

These nuts provide something different and special for a cocktail party or an evening of entertaining at home. Just watch the cashews carefully once they go into the oven, as you can wind up overtoasting (burning) them quite easily. Take it from me; I know from experience! MAKES 2 CUPS

2 cups raw cashews

3 or 4 fresh rosemary sprigs. roughly torn

1 teaspoon chili powder

1/4 teaspoon salt

1 tablespoon sugar

2 tablespoons canola oil

Couple dashes of cayenne

Preheat the oven to 375°F.

Combine all the ingredients in a large mixing bowl and toss together until the cashews are evenly and well coated. Turn the nuts out onto a foil-lined baking sheet and bake for about 10 minutes, until the cashews are lightly colored and fragrant. Set aside to cool before serving.

Whole Wheat Orzo, Mushroom, and Pecan "Risotto"

Not only is whole wheat orzo better for you, but I found it to have more flavor and texture. It gives off starch during the cooking process, lending the finished product a creaminess even though there is very little oil in the dish, no butter, and, of course, no rice. SERVES 4

---

3 tablespoons canola oil

1 medium onion, finely chopped

10 ounces cremini mushrooms, roughly chopped

1 teaspoon salt

1 teaspoon ground allspice

Freshly ground black pepper

2 cups whole wheat orzo

3 cups chicken or vegetable stock

Finely grated Parmesan cheese, for garnish

1 cup toasted pecan halves, crushed

Preheat the oven to 350°F.

In a 4-quart heavy-bottomed pot, heat the oil over medium-high heat. Add the onion, mushrooms, and salt. Cook, partially covered, stirring often, until the onion and mushrooms soften and the mushrooms give off their liquid, about 10 minutes. Then cook, uncovered, until nearly all of the liquid has evaporated, about 5 minutes longer. Stir in the allspice and pepper to taste and cook for a minute longer, just until fragrant. Mix in the orzo until it is thoroughly incorporated.

Add the stock, bring the mixture to a simmer, and then reduce the heat to medium-low and cook, partially covered, stirring often, until the orzo is *al dente* and the mixture resembles risotto in consistency, about 20 minutes. Ladle into serving bowls and top each serving with the grated Parmesan and a handful of the crushed pecans.

nut trivia

Not that you needed more convincing, but here are a few handy facts about nuts that you probably didn't know:

Eating just one cup of almonds provides you with your full daily dose of magnesium, which helps relax arteries and improves blood flow.

Just ten hazelnuts contain nearly half of the day's requirement of manganese, a trace mineral that helps protect cells from free radicals.

Walnuts contain high doses of compounds that fight inflammation, and cashews are bursting with bone- and skin-protecting copper.

What do peanuts have in common with red wine? They both contain resveratrol, the world-famous compound that's believed to give red wine many of its health benefits. Of course, peanuts contain small amounts of resveratrol compared with a typical glass of red wine. But then again, you can load up on peanuts and not wake up the next day with a hangover.

walnuts
almonds
peanuts
pecans
cashews
pine nuts
hazelnuts

Grilled Shrimp in Ajo Blanco

Ajo blanco is a traditional Spanish cold soup made primarily from almonds. The recipe requires blanched almonds rather than roasted almonds, which aren't milky enough. You should be able to find these blanched almonds at any large supermarket, health food store, or nut shop. SERVES 6

For the Shrimp:

10 ounces shrimp, peeled and deveined

½ teaspoon hot red pepper flakes

I teaspoon smoked paprika

2 tablespoons olive oil

Salt and freshly ground black pepper

For the Ajo Blanco:

6 ounces white country bread, crusts removed

2 cups ice water

I cup whole blanched almonds

3 tablespoons sherry vinegar or rice wine vinegar

2 garlic cloves, finely chopped

½ teaspoon Worcestershire sauce

½ teaspoon salt

¼ cup olive oil

For the Garnish:

Olive oil

Chopped parsley

Smoked paprika

To marinate the shrimp, combine the shrimp with the hot red pepper, paprika, olive oil, and salt and pepper to taste in a large resealable plastic bag. Marinate in the refrigerator for at least 30 minutes and up to overnight.

To make the *ajo blanco*, soak the bread in the ice water in a mixing bowl until the bread is soft and falling apart, about 10 minutes. Transfer the bread and water to a blender along with the almonds, vinegar, garlic, Worcestershire, and salt and blend until smooth. With the blender still on, gradually add the olive oil through the opening in the lid of the blender until fully incorporated and the mixture is thick and smooth. Store in the refrigerator until ready to serve.

Heat a cast-iron grill pan over high heat for about 5 minutes, until you can hold your hand about 4 inches from the pan's surface for no more than several seconds. Grill the shrimp until slightly blackened and just cooked through, about 3 minutes per side.

Pour the *ajo blanco* into serving bowls, top with a few of the cooked shrimp, and garnish with a drizzle of olive oil, some chopped parsley, and a dash of smoked paprika.

Roasted Red Pepper, Pine Nut, and Currant Relish

Serve this with a grilled meaty white fish like mahimahi, chicken, pork, or lamb. MAKES ABOUT 2 CUPS

---

2 large red bell peppers

2 tablespoons canola oil

1 small red onion, halved lengthwise and thinly sliced lengthwise

1 cup dried currants

¼ cup cider vinegar

¼ cup sugar

¾ cup pine nuts, lightly toasted and roughly chopped in a food processor

Salt

Preheat the broiler to its highest heat and position the top rack of the oven about 6 inches from the heat element.

Rub each pepper with a tablespoon of the oil and place on a foil-lined baking sheet. Broil the peppers, turning 3 or 4 times during the cooking, until blackened on all sides, 25 to 30 minutes in total. Transfer the blackened peppers to a small mixing bowl and cover tightly with plastic wrap. Allow the peppers to cool fully in the bowl; then remove the peppers, leaving any pepper liquid remaining at the bottom of the bowl.

Peel the blackened skins from the peppers, discard the stems and seeds, and cut the flesh of the peppers lengthwise into thin strips about ¼ inch thick. Return the sliced peppers to the original mixing bowl with the reserved pepper liquor.

Combine the onion, currants, vinegar, sugar, and 1 cup water in a large saucepan over medium-high heat. Bring to a simmer and continue cooking until nearly all the liquid has evaporated and the mixture is thick and jammy, about 25 minutes.

Remove the mixture from the heat, stir in the pine nuts and the sliced peppers with their juice, and season with salt to taste.

Chicken in Garam Masala–Spiced Cashew Cream

Garam masala is a spice mixture used in Indian food and found at most supermarkets. There is a good bit of cinnamon in it, which lends a sweet note and works well with the cashews. The creaminess of this dish comes not from dairy products but solely from the cashews. I find it is best served on top of a bed of brown basmati rice. SERVES 6

---

5 cups chicken stock

1 medium onion, roughly chopped

2 large garlic cloves, smashed

Juice of 1 lemon

One 2-inch piece fresh ginger, finely grated

5 fresh thyme sprigs, stems removed

¼ teaspoon cayenne

2 teaspoons garam masala

2 tablespoons honey

1 teaspoon salt

2 cups raw cashews

3 tablespoons tomato paste

1½ pounds skinless, boneless chicken breasts, cut into roughly 1-inch cubes

One 15-ounce can chickpeas, drained

Leaves from ½ bunch of fresh cilantro, finely chopped

Combine all the ingredients except the chicken and the chickpeas in a large saucepan. Bring to a simmer over medium-high heat and cook for 15 minutes. Remove from the heat and, working in batches, pour the sauce into a blender and blend until completely smooth and creamy. Return the sauce to the saucepan, add the cubed chicken and the chickpeas to the sauce, and bring the mixture to a simmer over medium heat. Cook, partially covered, for 15 minutes longer, stirring frequently.

Broiled Lamb Chops with Walnut and Mint Gremolata

Lamb is a staple in the Mediterranean diet, which Anahad uses as a reference point in many of our discussions about healthful eating, so it is only appropriate to include a lamb recipe or two in this book. Gremolata is traditionally made with just lemon zest, parsley, and garlic. It is also normally used to finish classic osso buco, so this is somewhat of a bastardization, but the addition of almonds makes for some nice texture, and the mint is a better pairing for lamb than the traditional parsley.

SERVES 4

For the Lamb Chops:

4 shoulder lamb chops (about 12 ounces each)

Salt and freshly ground black pepper

2 tablespoons olive oil

For the Gremolata:

1 cup raw walnuts

Leaves from 1 bunch of fresh mint, finely chopped

Grated zest of 1 lemon

3 garlic cloves, finely chopped

½ teaspoon salt

Freshly ground black pepper to taste

2 tablespoons olive oil

Preheat the broiler to high and adjust the oven rack so that it is about 6 inches from the broiler element.

Season the lamb chops generously with salt and pepper and evenly rub the olive oil over the meat. Place the lamb chops on a broiler pan and cook for 6 to 7 minutes per side for medium.

While the lamb is cooking, make the gremolata: Use a food processor to chop the walnuts to the consistency of very coarse sand. Transfer the ground walnuts to a large mixing bowl and mix in the remaining ingredients.

Top each lamb chop with a good sprinkling of the gremolata and serve.

Healthy Kung Pao Chicken

Kung pao chicken, despite its presence on every Chinese take-out menu in the country, is quite an authentic and traditional Chinese dish. This is a good reproduction of the kung pao you know and love, minus the MSG and maybe some other bad stuff. Be sure to use light soy sauce, or it will end up tasting too salty. If you're looking for something spicy, add in the teaspoon of hot red pepper flakes. Serve with brown rice. SERVES 6

For the Chicken and Marinade:

1 pound skinless, boneless chicken breast, cut into ¾-inch cubes

2 tablespoons light soy sauce

1 tablespoon rice wine vinegar

Freshly ground black pepper, to taste

For the Cooking Sauce:

2 tablespoons cornstarch

¼ cup light soy sauce

2 teaspoons black bean sauce

2 tablespoons oyster sauce

½ teaspoon dark sesame oil

2 tablespoons rice wine vinegar

1 tablespoon dark brown sugar

For the Stir Fry:

¼ cup canola oil

8 dried chiles de arból, broken in half

1 teaspoon hot red pepper flakes (optional)

2 large celery stalks, sliced on an angle about ¼ inch thick

6 ounces shiitake mushrooms, stems removed and caps thinly sliced

2 garlic cloves, minced

One 2-inch piece fresh ginger, finely grated

5 ounces sliced canned water chestnuts, drained

1 large bunch or 2 small bunches of scallions, sliced

1 cup unsalted peanuts, crushed

Combine the chicken with the marinade ingredients in a large mixing bowl. Stir well and set aside.

In another mixing bowl, whisk together the cornstarch and ¼ cup water; then whisk in the remaining sauce ingredients and set aside.

Prepare all the ingredients for the stir-fry and have them sitting at the ready.

Heat a large stainless-steel skillet or traditional wok over the highest heat for about 3 minutes. Add the oil, and as soon as the oil begins to smoke, add the marinated chicken and distribute the chicken evenly in the pan. Move the chicken around the pan nearly constantly until the chicken is a dark golden brown on all sides, about 4 minutes. Use a slotted metal spoon to remove the chicken from the pan, discard all but about 3 table-spoons of the oil, and return the pan to the heat.

Add the chiles to the pan and stir them around until they turn a dark brick color all over, just a minute or two, then add the hot red pepper flakes if you want the dish spicy, along with the celery and shiitake mushrooms, and cook the vegetables, stirring constantly, until they soften, 2 to 3 minutes. Stir in the garlic and ginger, and as soon as it is fragrant, add the water chestnuts, reserved cooking sauce, and reserved browned chicken pieces. Cook the mixture, stirring constantly, until thick and glossy, about 4 minutes. Add half of the scallions and half of the peanuts and cook for 1 minute longer.

Pour the kung pao into a large serving dish, sprinkle with the remaining scallions and peanuts, and serve family-style with sides of brown rice.

Grandma Bernice's Almond Lemon Sponge Cake

This sponge cake is a version of my grandmother Bernice's beloved recipe. I never met my grandmother, but my father has kept a piece of her alive by making a batch of her cakes every year. The original recipe uses matzo meal and potato starch, but those ingredients can be hard to find sometimes, so I've adjusted the recipe to use whole wheat flour and cornstarch. This makes a slightly denser, chewier cake, but the result is still close enough that I think I can rightly attribute it to my grandmother. SERVES 12

I cup raw almonds

½ cup whole wheat flour

¼ cup cornstarch

9 large eggs. separated

½ teaspoon salt

Juice and grated zest of 1½ lemons (about ⅓ cup juice)

¼ cup room-temperature water

1⅓ cups sugar

Preheat the oven to 350°F.

Use a food processor to grind the almonds to the consistency of very coarse sand. Whisk together the flour and cornstarch and reserve.

Use a stand mixer fitted with the whisk attachment to whip the egg whites and salt to soft peaks. Do not overbeat the egg whites or the cake will turn out dry.

Set the egg whites aside, switch to a paddle attachment, and in a separate bowl beat the yolks until thick, creamy, and pale yellow, about 5 minutes.

Combine the lemon juice, lemon zest, and water. Then gradually add the sugar to the beaten yolks and beat until incorporated and the mixture thickens. Alternately add the lemon juice mixture and the dry mixture. Finally, beat in the ground almonds.

Use a round-handled wooden spoon to fold the yolk mixture into the whites until fully incorporated. Pour the batter into an ungreased 10-inch angel food cake tube pan and bake for about 50 minutes, until the top of the cake is golden brown and a wooden skewer inserted into the middle of the cake comes out clean.

Remove the cake from the oven and immediately turn it upside down to cool fully in the pan, about 2 hours.

walnuts and sleep

Spend most of your days chasing those elusive Zs?

If you've got sleeping problems, walnuts might give you a little boost. Studies show that walnuts are high in melatonin, a hormone that helps regulate the sleep cycle. It's also widely used as a sleep aid and remedy for jet lag. But unfortunately, humans produce less and less of it as they age.

Walnuts may be one way to stem the loss of this vital hormone. Eating just a small amount of walnuts has been shown in studies at the University of Texas to raise levels of melatonin in the blood threefold.

Other studies have shown that taking melatonin two hours before bedtime can dramatically improve sleep.

Next time you're suffering from a bout of insomnia, you might want to reach for a bag of walnuts before you start counting sheep.

walnuts
almonds
peanuts
pecans
cashews
pine nuts
hazelnuts

Pecan Mini-Meringues

These little meringues are crisp without being fall-apart dry, so you can still really appreciate the texture of the chopped pecans. They are so simple that every flavor shines through. MAKES ABOUT 15 MERINGUES

3 egg whites, at room temperature

¼ teaspoon salt

¾ cup sugar

½ teaspoon vanilla extract

¼ teaspoon ground cinnamon

2 cups pecan halves, roughly chopped

Preheat the oven to 200°F.

Using a stand mixer fitted with the whisk attachment, whisk the egg whites and salt to soft peaks. Beat in the sugar ¼ cup at a time, allowing a minute or so between additions. Once all the sugar has been incorporated, add the vanilla and cinnamon and beat the mixture for about 5 minutes longer, until thick and glossy.

Fold the pecans into the egg white mixture and spoon onto a cookie sheet lined with wax paper to form meringues 2 to 3 inches in diameter.

Bake for 1½ hours, until the meringues are dry and crisp. Allow to cool fully before serving.

Flourless Hazelnut and Dark Chocolate Torte

There's no doubt about it: this is a decadent dessert. But there is no processed flour in the recipe at all, and the two central ingredients—hazelnuts and dark chocolate—are both rich in heart-healthy fats and antioxidants. MAKES ONE 9-INCH CAKE, SERVING 8 TO 9

I cup blanched hazelnuts

8 ounces bittersweet chocolate (at least 60% cacao)

¼ cup canola oil

3 tablespoons butter

6 eggs, separated

¼ teaspoon salt

½ cup dark brown sugar

¼ cup granulated sugar

I teaspoon vanilla extract

2 tablespoons Dutch-process cocoa

Preheat the oven to 325°F. Grease a 9-inch springform pan and line the bottom of the pan with parchment.

Finely grind the hazelnuts in a food processor until they reach a coarse, sandy consistency.

Either in the microwave or in a double boiler over hot water, melt the chocolate with the oil and butter, stirring together to form a homogenous mixture. Set aside in a warm place.

With a stand mixer fitted with the whisk attachment, beat the egg whites and salt to soft peaks and set aside. Switch to the paddle attachment and, in a separate bowl, beat the egg yolks, sugars, and vanilla extract on medium-high speed until thick and creamy, about 5 minutes. Reduce the speed of the mixer to low and add the chocolate and butter mixture, then the cocoa powder. Fold in the whipped egg whites until smooth.

Pour into a greased and parchment-lined 9-inch springform pan and bake for 45 to 50 minutes, just until a wooden skewer inserted into the center of the cake comes out clean.

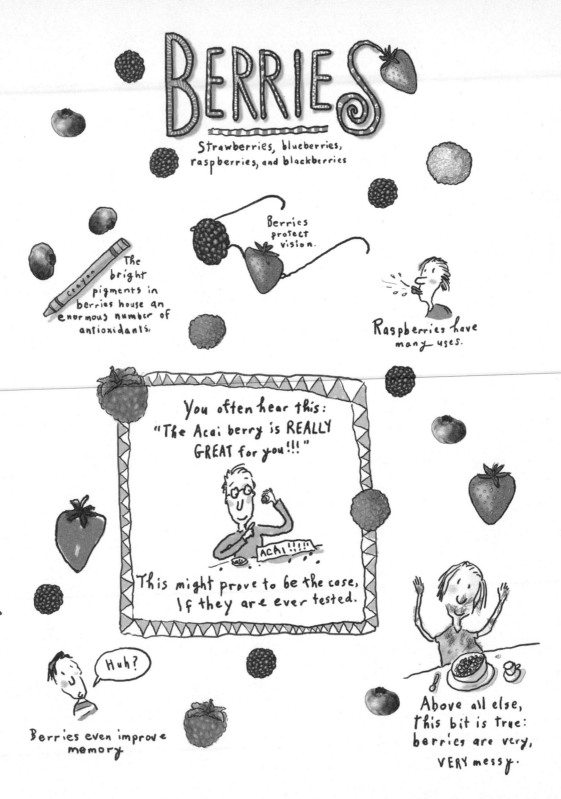

10

BERRIES

Walk into any health food store and you'll be bombarded by labels trying to grab your attention with buzzwords tempting you to shell out your hard-earned cash for a miracle elixir. Today the buzzword most savvy marketers have learned to rely on should come as no surprise. It's the word you often see in a bold or fluorescent font (perhaps with an exclamation point too) as you make your way down the store aisles: *antioxidants*.

A decade ago, no one gave them any thought. But now all that has changed. The word is on the lips of every health-conscious American, and the food and supplement industries are eager to capitalize, slapping antioxidant labels on a rapidly growing number of products with bloated price tags.

The hoopla is hard to ignore. According to Nielsen, sales of foods promoted as antioxidant-rich ballooned by 11 percent in 2008, reaching a staggering $1.9 billion, while pricey antioxidant supplements brought in even more.

Products made with acai berries are at the top of the list—the market has been flooded with more than fifty products with the stuff. But while this purplish fruit from the Brazilian rain forest has been touted as an anti-inflammatory, anticancer, antioxidant-laden ambrosia, it has yet to undergo a single human trial. About the only thing we know for sure is that it contains plenty of anti-oxidants.

But what is all the fuss about antioxidants anyway?

Quite simply, they protect our bodies from the devastating effects of oxygen. As ironic as it sounds, the very air that we breathe and the oxygen it contains gives us life but can also take it away. This happens bit by bit, as highly reactive by-products of oxygen circulate in our bloodstreams and claw at our cells and the DNA within them, ultimately contributing to everything from Alzheimer's to cancer to heart disease and the very process of aging itself.

We need a strong line of defense to stop this from happening, and that's where antioxidants come in (hence the name). They have the power to sweep away the free radicals that would otherwise do their dirty work with abandon, which is why you want plenty of them circulating in your system.

You could accomplish this by going out and spending forty bucks on a bottle of acai. Perhaps it's worth it; but perhaps it's not. Scientists just don't know yet.

On the other hand, you could turn to a much cheaper, proven alternative—one that is about good old-fashioned berries, grown right here in North America. Blueber-ries. Blackberries. Strawberries. And, of course, raspberries. This is your all-star team of superfruits. These are four berries that you definitely want to have in your diet. Loaded with nutrients, they've been shown in studies to help protect against everything from heart disease to memory loss.

The acai berry's claim to fame is its enormous level of antioxidants. But researchers in Spain and Brazil collected a variety of fruits and measured their antioxidant capaci-ties as part of a 2006 study, and acai berries were topped by none other than strawber-ries. Blueberries, raspberries, and blackberries are right up there as well when it comes to antioxidants—especially blackberries, which one study in 2006 ranked at the top of a list of more than a thousand foods commonly available in the United States. And when the USDA analyzed a hundred fruits and vegetables for antioxidant content in 2004, strawberries, blackberries, raspberries, and blueberries crowned their list as well (for comparison's sake, a single cup of blueberries has three times the amount of an-tioxidants as a single Gala apple and about four times the amount of a navel orange).

One of the best approaches to good health, research shows, is to eat a rainbow of fruits and vegetables. That's because the bright and beautiful colors in the berry family are about more than just aesthetics. The eye-pleasing pigments that give fruits and vegetables their colors are powerful antioxidants, capable of vacuuming away the free radicals (many of them by-products of oxygen) that are so hazardous to health. So when I see Dave's hands stained a brilliant shade of blue after an afternoon of cooking with blueberries, or the crimson ink on our kitchen countertop after I've rinsed a batch or two of raspberries, I'm reminded just how potent these little guys are.

Berries surely seemed like an antioxidant home run, but we figured we'd talk to someone who knows antioxidants better than anyone.

Dr. Jim Joseph spends his time studying free radicals and the foods that can stop or reverse the destruction that these pernicious little molecules can wreak. Naturally, berries are one of his main areas of research. As director of the neuroscience lab at the USDA human nutrition research center on aging at Tufts University, Dr. Joseph has become something of a cheerleader for berries. You won't find anyone more enthusiastic about these little bundles of nutrition. That was evident from our very first exchange, when Dr. Joseph—with a little good humor—showed just how much time he spends pondering the berry.

"So, Dr. Joseph, exactly how healthy *are* these berries?"

"Well," he told me, "I'll put it this way: They're pretty amazing. You have to be careful with berries. They'll turn you into a conservative."

I paused for a moment, scratching my head before I finally asked: "A conservative? Ah, come again?"

"They'll turn you into a lib-*berr*-tarian," he shot back, letting out a sly laugh.

Keep in mind: for a scientist, that's pretty edgy humor.

But what we talked about next was hardly a joke. Having studied antioxidants and berries for years, Dr. Joseph was blunt and plainspoken as he got down to the facts.

"As you age," he explained, "you get less able to deal with these very reactive molecules called *free radicals*. So the idea is to add things to your diet to make yourself less vulnerable to oxidative stress and its evil twin of aging, inflammation. Every so-called major killer that people talk about in books, newspapers, and the media—heart disease, Alzheimer's, Parkinson's, diabetes, you name it—has an oxidative stress and an inflammatory component. Most of these diseases increase in frequency as a function of age. And so the idea is to get more things in your diet that are high in antioxidants and anti-inflammatory agents. One of the best ways to do that, without a doubt, is with berries. They all have different properties, but mainly they're extremely good antioxidants and anti-inflammatories."

Dr. Joseph elaborated that berries contain a group of anti-inflammatory compounds that act as painkillers; they are called COX-2 inhibitors, a term you probably recognize. You may recall that COX-2 inhibitors are so effective—in some cases even more so than ibuprofen—that they were sold as the blockbuster prescription drugs Celebrex, Vioxx, and Bextra. But berries have a distinct advantage.

"Berries contain COX-2 inhibitors—only without all the dangerous side effects," Dr. Joseph said.

Of course, no one is suggesting turning to berries to replace prescription drugs. The point is that most people have no idea how many impressive nutrients Mother Nature has crammed inside those colorful little packages.

The best way to consume these four superberries is to view them as the four wheels of a car: Each very similar, but unique in its own way. And each is equally indispensable. Each has its own assortment of antioxidants and nutrients, and a combination of all four creates the best results. That's not to say you need to eat them all simultaneously—otherwise I'm sure researchers would be hard at work right now trying to come up with some scary mutant hybrid berry with a name like *strawblackblasberry*—it only means that you should include all of them in your diet with equal weight.

Strawberries, for example, are a good source of potassium, a mineral that your cells need to help convert carbohydrates into energy. Without enough of this mineral your muscles wouldn't twitch and your heart wouldn't tick. Nor would your brain be able to process the words on this page. According to the Institute of Medicine, proper intake of potassium can help ward off hypertension and reduce the risk of stroke, and yet the average American typically consumes less than half the recommended daily amount. Adding strawberries to your diet is one surefire way to help you hit the mark.

With blueberries you get a hearty dose of fiber (especially soluble fiber, the kind that keeps you fuller longer), an abundance of antioxidants, and even a little resveratrol, the life-extending compound that revealed red wine as a health food. With raspberries there's vitamin C, the ammunition you need to keep your immune system in shape, shorten colds, and maintain optimal health. A single cup of raspberries packs more than half your daily requirement of vitamin C. Then there are blackberries, containing everything from protein to vitamin E and even omega-3 fatty acids.

How's that for a starting lineup? And fortunately, berries are no bitter pill to swallow. As Dave puts it:

Maybe berries are so good because Mother Nature wanted to make sure there was no way we could turn them down. How's that for intelligent design! I mean, berries are more like a treat for me than anything else. If someone told me I had to eat beautifully ripe raspberries for the rest of my days, I'd be laughing all the way to the berry bowl! Berries and chocolate. Berries and cream. That is the stuff dreams are made of—and some racy ones at that!

In making up a recipe-testing schedule for the book, I purposefully saved the berry chapter until the end because I knew what a simple pleasure it would be for me to develop berry recipes. The thought of cooking (and eating!) all those berries was something that kept me excited for months. And the reality lived up to my expectations.

I used berries in new ways—whether it was roasting blackberries with pork or combining blueberries and smoked fish—and the berries never let me down. Most people think of berries as a dessert food or nothing more than a sweet garnish, but I find berries can be much more versatile and sophisticated than that. Sure, they are absolutely fantastic as a sweet treat, but what makes berries so flexible is the fact that they toe the line between sweet and tart, juicy yet fibrous, so they can play in the savory realm as well as in the sweet one. Anahad had a hard time coming around to this fact (or maybe the blueberry and smoked trout combination was a bit of an intense introduction), but even he quickly turned the corner and was soon looking out for the next savory berry dish to come out of the kitchen.

Balsamic Berry Salad with Arugula, Goat Cheese, and Sunflower Seeds

The natural tartness of the berries is a good foil for the creaminess of the goat cheese. The sunflower seeds add some nice texture but, because of their mild flavor, don't impede full enjoyment of the flavor of the berries.

SERVES 4 TO 6

½ cup balsamic vinegar

1 pound strawberries, hulled and sliced lengthwise about ¼ inch thick

6 ounces fresh raspberries

2 tablespoons finely chopped fresh chives

2 ounces mild creamy goat cheese, crumbled

¼ cup raw sunflower seeds

2 ounces baby arugula

About 15 fresh basil leaves, roughly chopped

3 tablespoons olive oil

Juice of ½ lemon

Salt and freshly cracked black pepper

Heat the vinegar in a small, heavy-bottomed saucepan over medium heat and simmer until reduced by half, about 10 minutes. Remove from the heat and set aside to cool.

Combine the strawberries, raspberries, and chives in a large mixing bowl. Pour the cool balsamic reduction into the bowl; then toss to incorporate well. Add the crumbled goat cheese and sunflower seeds and toss once very gently.

Combine the arugula and basil in a separate mixing bowl and toss with the olive oil and lemon juice. Season lightly with the salt.

To serve, arrange a heap of the arugula salad on each plate and top with the berry mixture. Finish with some of the cracked pepper on top.

strawberry and raspberry
for eyesight

We've all heard the old bromide about eating carrots to boost your vision. But it turns out that mothers may need to promote something else when it comes to protecting eyesight.

Or at least that's what researchers at Harvard Medical School and Brigham and Women's Hospital have found. In a large 2004 study, they looked at more than 110,000 people and their diets, trying to find out whether certain vegetables, fruits, or vitamins could help ward off deteriorating eyesight. They found that a person's intake of vegetables and vitamins didn't make much difference, but eating three or more servings a day of fruits like berries helped lower the risk of diseases that damage vision.

You won't find any carrots in our berry salad. But you will find a couple servings of raspberries and strawberries, which give all new meaning to the phrase *eye-pleasing*.

using berries year-round

In this day and age, there's no reason you can't incorporate berries into your diet year-round.

In temperate climates, berries are really in season only in summer, but between the farmers in places like California, Mexico, and South America, you can find fresh berries on the super-market shelf virtually any time of year. These berries are usually lacking that certain summertime *je ne sais quoi,* and if you're worried about your carbon footprint they probably aren't the best option anyway. In a pinch, though, it's a real luxury to have them at your disposal.

When berries aren't in season or come in from California looking pretty grim, I turn to frozen berries. Frozen berries have the advantage of being picked and pre-served at the proper ripeness; they are often less expensive than fresh berries out of season; and while they aren't great for all applications, there is no shortage of ways to make good use of them.

So my berry motto: "Buy fresh when berries are in season." Otherwise, take advantage of the frozen ones.

Watercress, Wheat Berry, and Potato Salad with Blackberries

Wheat berries need to be soaked overnight and then cooked for about an hour before they take on a really pleasant chewiness. I particularly love the texture of them in this salad because the combination of the soft blackberry flesh, the slight crunchiness from the blackberry seeds, and the playful bounce of the wheat berries is kind of like having a fun circus on your palate. SERVES 6

For the Salad:

3 cups presoaked wheat berries

3 ounces watercress

6 ounces blackberries

8 ounces baby white potatoes, steamed until tender and halved

4 ounces imported feta cheese, crumbled

For the Dressing:

1 large shallot, finely chopped

2 teaspoons whole-grain mustard

3 tablespoons red wine vinegar

¼ cup canola oil

¼ teaspoon salt

Freshly ground black pepper to taste

In a large pot, bring 4 to 5 quarts of salted water to a boil over high heat. Add the wheat berries, cover loosely, and reduce the heat to medium. Simmer the wheat berries for about an hour, until they are tender but still a bit chewy. Strain the wheat berries and set aside to dry and cool.

Combine the dressing ingredients in a sealable container and shake until smooth.

When the wheat berries are cool, toss them with the other salad ingredients in a large mixing bowl. Pour the dressing over the top of the salad ingredients and toss well.

what berries might do for you:
a scientific breakdown

Here's a quick rundown of interesting and pretty compelling studies done recently on incorporating berries into your diet.

An eight-week study by Finnish researchers in 2008 found that people who ate a cup of berries a day lowered their systolic blood pressure (the top number in your blood pressure reading) by as much as seven points and increased their HDL cholesterol (the good kind) an average of 5.2 percent.

A study by British researchers in 2008 found that a cup of blueberries a day for twelve weeks improved working memory.

Also in 2008, Ohio State scientists found that in patients with a high risk of colon cancer, those who were given black raspberry extract developed up to 59 percent fewer polyps than those given a placebo.

A 1995 study of nearly fifty thousand men by researchers at Harvard Medical School found that regular consumption of strawberries was "significantly associated with lower prostate cancer risk."

Blueberry, Wax Bean, and Smoked Trout Salad

When I told Anahad about my plan for this salad, he looked at me somewhat in disbelief. "Dude, blueberries and smoked fish? What are you thinking?" His reaction gave me pause, but my blueberry and smoked fish combination and I finally prevailed. And in the end, of course, Anahad was coming back for seconds. SERVES 6

1 pound wax beans, trimmed

8 ounces smoked trout, skin removed

1 shallot, minced

⅓ cup thick Greek-style yogurt

Juice of 1 lemon

2 tablespoons olive oil

2 teaspoons whole-grain mustard

1 pint fresh blueberries

Leaves from 1 large bunch of celery

2 large celery stalks, halved lengthwise and thinly sliced crosswise

Freshly ground black pepper

Place the wax beans in a large microwave-safe bowl, cover with a tight-fitting lid or plate, and microwave on high until the beans are cooked but still a bit snappy, just a couple minutes. Remove the cover and set aside to cool.

Use a couple small forks or your fingers to flake the trout into bite-sized chunks.

Whisk the shallot, yogurt, lemon juice, olive oil, and mustard together in a large mixing bowl. Add the beans, blueberries, trout, celery leaves, and sliced celery. Toss well and season with pepper to taste.

Roasted Pork Loin with Port, Prunes, and Blackberries

A pork loin roast is one of the most lean and tender cuts you can get your hands on. I love pairing the flavor of pork with sweet elements, so the blackberries with prunes and port were a natural fit for me. When you present this on a large platter and garnish with fresh blackberries and rosemary sprigs, this dish also makes for the perfect elegant entrée for a small dinner party. SERVES 6

For the Roast:

2½ pounds pork loin roast

¼ cup olive oil

2 teaspoons kosher salt

Freshly ground black pepper to taste

4 fresh rosemary sprigs

6 large garlic cloves, smashed

About 20 whole cloves

For the Sauce:

1 cup tawny port

1 cup chicken stock

2 tablespoons good balsamic vinegar

2 star anise

20 prunes

6 ounces blackberries

Preheat the oven to 350°F.

Place the roast in a large resealable bag and add the remaining ingredients. Seal the bag, massage the marinade ingredients into the meat, and refrigerate overnight.

Remove the roast from the refrigerator and let stand at room temperature for about an hour before cooking.

Place the roast in a foil-lined roasting dish, leaving the marinade ingredients behind in the plastic bag.

Roast the pork loin for about 40 minutes. While the roast is cooking, combine the port, stock, balsamic vinegar, star anise, and prunes in a saucepan and bring to a simmer. After the roast has cooked for 40 minutes, pour the sauce over the roast, toss on half of the blackberries, and roast for 15 minutes longer.

Transfer the roast to a cutting board and allow to rest about 10 minutes; then slice the roast into ½-inch slices.

To serve, arrange the slices on a platter and top with the juices and fruit left in the pan. Garnish with sprigs of rosemary and the other half of the fresh blackberries.

pork as a meaty protein

A pork loin roast is very lean meat and still one of the most tender cuts you can find at the butcher. It's a great option if you want meaty lean protein that isn't chicken or fish. When most Americans go to make a family roast, you'll likely find them reaching for a hunk of beef. Don't get me wrong, I love beef as much as the next guy, and a beef tenderloin would be incredibly delicious in our pork loin recipe, but a quick look at the numbers reveals it has twice the total fat for the same serving size.

Seared Salmon with Blackberry Sauce and Olive Oil–Braised Fennel

The first rule that people hear when they're learning about wine is that red wine goes with meat and white wine goes with fish. But those are just the guidelines, and I love eating some meatier fish with red wine, particularly salmon, which is why I thought of this combination here. The strained sauce makes for an elegant presentation. SERVES 4

For the Fennel:

1 small fennel bulb, cored, stalks removed, fronds reserved, and bulb thinly sliced lengthwise

¼ cup olive oil

Salt

For the Sauce:

1 large shallot, thinly sliced

1 garlic clove, smashed

1½ cups red wine

1½ cups chicken stock

1 tablespoon plus 1 teaspoon sugar

3 fresh thyme sprigs

12 ounces fresh blackberries

2 teaspoons cornstarch

For the Salmon:

2 tablespoons canola oil

About 1½ pounds salmon (preferably wild), cut into 4 equal fillets

Salt and freshly ground black pepper

Combine the fennel and olive oil in a small, heavy-bottomed saucepan over medium heat and cook, partially covered, stirring occasionally, until the fennel is very tender, sweet, and very lightly browned, about 20 minutes. Season with salt to taste and keep warm.

Combine all the ingredients for the sauce, except the cornstarch, in a heavy-bottomed saucepan and bring to a simmer over medium heat. Simmer until the berries are so soft that they fall apart easily with just the slightest prodding with a fork and the mixture is reduced by about half, roughly 30 minutes.

Set a fine-mesh sieve over the top of a large bowl. Pour the berry mixture into the sieve and use a spoon to strain the sauce through the sieve, firmly pressing and stirring the solids until as much liquid has been extracted as possible. Discard the solids and transfer the strained sauce back to the saucepan. Put the cornstarch in a small bowl and add a couple tablespoons of the strained sauce to the cornstarch. Stir until homogenous and then add the cornstarch to the saucepan and cook over medium heat, whisking constantly, until the mixture thickens, 4 to 5 minutes. Remove from the heat but keep warm.

To prepare the fish, heat the oil in a large nonstick skillet over medium-high heat. Season the salmon fillets generously with salt and pepper. Cook on both sides until golden brown and cooked through, 4 to 5 minutes per side.

To serve, spoon a couple tablespoons of the sauce onto each serving plate. Top with a portion of the braised fennel and a piece of salmon on top of that. Garnish with a fennel frond.

blueberries as bacteria killer?

You've probably heard the old saw about cranberries having antibacterial properties. The reason, according to studies, is that they contain high levels of proanthocyanidin, an antioxidant that prevents *E. coli* from adhering to cells that line the urinary tract. Studies have found that these compounds help lower the risk of urinary infections, which is where the widespread old wives' tale comes from.

But blueberries have the same properties and very similar results. According to the USDA, cranberries are extremely high in proanthocyanidins, but the proanthocyanidin content of blueberries is about 80 percent. And ounce for ounce, blueberries contain far more than you'll find in bottled cranberry juice. So the next time you want a little antibacterial boost from cranberries, remember the blueberry.

Raspberry Soy Milk Ice Cream

It might seem odd to have a recipe for ice cream in a health-oriented cookbook, but this is a healthy ice cream alternative. Soy milk subs in for cream and milk here, but the texture of soy milk is so creamy that it results in a nice smooth texture. Adding a little thick Greek-style yogurt and plenty of honey helps too. Look for soy milk that is made from only soy milk and water and no thickeners like carageenan or guar gum.

SERVES 8

---

1 quart unsweetened soy milk

⅔ cup honey

2 teaspoons vanilla extract

⅓ cup thick Greek style yogurt

2 cups frozen raspberries

Combine the soy milk, honey, and vanilla in a large saucepan and heat for about 5 minutes, stirring frequently to dissolve the sugar into the soy milk. Remove from the heat, add the yogurt and raspberries, and transfer the mixture to a blender and, in batches if necessary, blend until smooth.

Turn on your ice cream maker and slowly pour the smooth soy milk and raspberry mixture into the machine; churn until it has the consistency of soft-serve ice cream, about 45 minutes. Immediately pour into a large sealable container, press plastic wrap onto the surface of the ice cream, seal the container, and freeze for at least several hours.

Remove from the freezer and let stand for 10 minutes before scooping.

Ricotta Cheesecake with Strawberry, Raspberry, and Rhubarb Compote

While this cheesecake falls squarely into the dessert category for its sugar and fat content, it's way healthier than any other cheesecake you're going to get your hands on, and it is absolutely delicious! It is probably my favorite sweet thing in the book, but without the berry and rhubarb compote, it really would be only half as good. And contrary to what you might have heard, you don't have to peel rhubarb. I never do, because the peel is where all the wonderful color is. SERVES 12

For the Crust:

6 graham crackers

½ cup dark brown sugar

½ teaspoon ground cinnamon

4 tablespoons (½ stick) butter, melted

For the Filling:

3 cups fresh ricotta cheese

8 ounces reduced-fat cream cheese, softened

½ cup granulated sugar

2 teaspoons vanilla extract

2 eggs

2 egg yolks

For the Compote:

8 ounces rhubarb

8 ounces fresh or frozen whole strawberries

6 ounces fresh or frozen whole raspberries

Juice of 1 lemon

¼ cup sugar

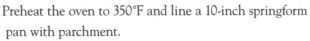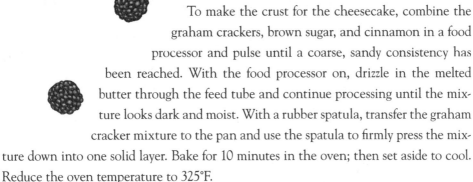

Preheat the oven to 350°F and line a 10-inch springform pan with parchment.

To make the crust for the cheesecake, combine the graham crackers, brown sugar, and cinnamon in a food processor and pulse until a coarse, sandy consistency has been reached. With the food processor on, drizzle in the melted butter through the feed tube and continue processing until the mixture looks dark and moist. With a rubber spatula, transfer the graham cracker mixture to the pan and use the spatula to firmly press the mixture down into one solid layer. Bake for 10 minutes in the oven; then set aside to cool. Reduce the oven temperature to 325°F.

While the crust is cooling, make the filling for the cake. Combine the ricotta, cream cheese (several seconds in the microwave will soften it), granulated sugar, vanilla, eggs, and egg yolks in a large mixing bowl. Use a whisk to whip all the ingredients together until a homogenous, creamy consistency is reached.

Once the springform pan is cool enough to handle again, wrap it up completely and tightly with a double layer of 2 separate sheets of extra-wide aluminum foil (to keep any water from leaking into the cake while it is baking). Set the foil-wrapped pan in a 12-inch, stainless-steel skillet or a baking dish large enough to hold the pan.

Pour the ricotta–cream cheese filling into the springform pan and smooth the top. Set the skillet or baking dish on the middle rack of the oven and pour boiling water three-quarters of the way up the side of the cake pan.

Bake for 1½ hours; then remove the cake pan from the water bath, dry it, remove the foil, and allow the cake to cool completely.

Once the cake has cooled completely, cover it with a piece of plastic wrap, transfer it to the refrigerator, and refrigerate for at least 2 hours but preferably overnight.

Make the compote by combining all the compote ingredients in a medium saucepan over medium heat. Heat until mixture has turned syrupy, the berries are soft, and the rhubarb has broken down, about 10 to 15 minutes. Transfer the compote to a container and set aside to cool before refrigerating until cold.

Slice the cheesecake with a sharp knife moistened with warm water and serve with a couple big spoonfuls of the compote over the top.

Blueberry, Lemon, and Olive Oil Cake with Smashed Blueberry Sauce

Frozen blueberries (and all frozen berries for that matter) are a wonderful thing because they give you access to ripe berries, at a decent price, at any time of year. Because they sort of turn to mush when they thaw out, they're really good for only certain applications like smoothies and certain kinds of baking. Enter this blueberry cake. Olive oil is the only fat here, but it's as rich as any pound cake. The slight bite of the olive oil is offset by the sweetness of the sugar and berries and the bright tanginess of the lemon. MAKES ONE 10-INCH BUNDT CAKE AND ABOUT 1½ CUPS OF BLUEBERRY SAUCE

For the Cake:

1 cup all-purpose flour

1 cup whole wheat flour

½ teaspoon fine salt

2 teaspoons baking powder

1 cup sugar

2 teaspoons vanilla extract

Grated zest of 1 lemon

Juice of ½ lemon

1 cup olive oil

3 eggs, at room temperature

8 ounces frozen blueberries

For the Blueberry Sauce:

8 ounces frozen blueberries

Juice of ½ lemon

½ cup sugar

Butter for the pan

Preheat the oven to 350°F. Butter a 10-inch Bundt pan.

To make the cake, whisk the flours, salt, baking powder, and sugar together in a large mixing bowl.

Using a stand mixer fitted with the paddle attachment, beat the vanilla, lemon zest, lemon juice, and the olive oil at medium-high speed until the mixture is light and creamy, about 4 minutes. Reduce the mixer speed to medium-low and add the eggs one at a time, waiting for each egg to incorporate fully before adding the next.

Reduce the mixer speed to low and gradually add the dry ingredients, beating just until fully incorporated. Then stir in the frozen blueberries.

Pour the batter into the Bundt pan and bake for 1 hour, until the top of the cake is golden brown and a knife or wooden skewer inserted into the middle of the cake comes out clean. Allow the cake to cool completely before turning it out and slicing.

While the cake is baking, make the blueberry sauce: Combine the blueberries, lemon juice, and sugar in a small saucepan over medium heat. Bring the mixture to a simmer and cook, using a fork to smash down the blueberries as they soften, until only blueberry chunks remain and the mixture has thickened, about 15 minutes.

To serve, slice the cake and top each slice with a couple good spoonfuls of the berry sauce.

Mixed-Berry Bread Pudding

My colleague Ben Mims, who is a fantastic baker, introduced me to a version of this dessert. Ironically there's no baking involved, but the result is as impressive as any one of his baked desserts. This was another opportunity to use lots of frozen berries, which adds a little flexibility when berries aren't in season, but if you have loads of fresh, delicious berries, you should, of course, use those instead. SERVES 12

26 ounces frozen mixed berries (strawberries, raspberries, blueberries, and blackberries)

⅔ cup honey

½ cup brandy

3 tablespoons crème de cassis, plus more for garnish

One 1½-pound loaf country white bread

Thick Greek-style yogurt

Fresh mint leaves for garnish

Combine the frozen berries, honey, brandy, and crème de cassis over medium heat in a large saucepan and heat gently, stirring frequently, until a loose, almost syrupy mixture is formed but the berries are still intact, about 7 minutes. Remove the berry mixture from the heat and set aside to cool.

Use a serrated knife to remove the crusts from the bread loaf and cut the bread into ⅓-inch slices.

Once the berry mixture has cooled to room temperature, begin to assemble the pudding. Coat the bottom of a 4-quart glass bowl with a ladle of the berry mixture, being sure to include several whole berries, since this will form the top of the dessert when you turn it out. Use a few bread slices to cover this first layer of berry mixture. Cover the first bread layer with a couple more ladles of the berry mixture; then cover with more bread slices. Repeat until all the bread and berry mixture has been used up, finishing with the berry mixture to saturate the last layer of bread.

Press a large sheet of plastic wrap over the final layer and then set a plate that is nearly the same size as the bowl opening on top of the plastic wrap. Weight the plate down with 2 large cans of tomatoes and refrigerate the pudding overnight.

When ready to serve, remove the cans, plate, and plastic wrap from the pudding. Run a knife along the sides of the pudding to loosen it from the bowl. Place a large serving plate over the top of the bowl and hold it firmly against the rim of the bowl as you quickly invert the bowl to turn out the pudding.

Slice the pudding into wedges and serve with dollops of yogurt, a drizzle of crème de cassis, and some fresh mint leaves.

ricotta rocks!

Anyone who knows cheese knows that no two are the same. Ricotta is no exception, particularly when it comes to nutrition.

Ricotta is creamy, lush, and even a little sweet. And unlike most cheeses, it's low in fat and high in a special type of protein, called *whey*. In fact, ricotta is technically not really a cheese at all. It's made from the liquid that's left over after the milkfat and proteins have been removed from milk during the process of making cheeses like mozzarella and provolone. That liquid is then "recooked," hence the name *ricotta*.

Because of the way it's made, fresh ricotta is naturally low in fat, typically less than 10 percent. But perhaps just as important is the fact that ricotta is such a great source of whey, one of the most high-quality proteins you can find—loaded with essential amino acids and an extremely effective fat burner and muscle builder.

Of all known proteins, whey has the highest biological value, which is simply a measure of how well your body absorbs and makes use of a particular type of protein. Whey ranks in with a value of 104, ahead of eggs (about 100) and even beef (80).

With ricotta, you get the most protein and fewest calories, making it a great substitute for other cheeses wherever possible. That's why we've added it to our light but tasty cheesecake, topped off with a hefty dose of berries. More flavor, less guilt. You can't really go wrong.

NOTES

1 Tomatoes

Gallus S, Tavani A, La Vecchia C.
Pizza and risk of acute myocardial infarction.
Eur J Clin Nutr. 2004 Nov; 58(11):1543–6.

Sesso HD, Liu S, Gaziano JM, Buring JE.
Dietary lycopene, tomato-based food products and cardiovascular disease
    in women.
J Nutr. 2003 Jul; 133(7):2336–41.

Gallus S, Bosetti C, et al.
Does pizza protect against cancer?
Int J Cancer. 2003 Nov 1; 107(2):283–4.

Willcox JK, et al.
Tomatoes and cardiovascular health.
Crit Rev Food Sci Nutr 2003; 43(1):1–18.

Etminan M, et al.
The role of tomato products and lycopene in the prevention of prostate cancer: A
    meta-analysis of observational studies.
Cancer Epidemiol Biomarkers Prev. 2004 Mar; 13(3):340–5.

Boileau TW, Liao Z, et al.
Prostate carcinogenesis in N-methyl-N-nitrosourea (NMU)-testosterone-treated rats fed tomato
powder, lycopene, or energy-restricted diets.
J Natl Cancer Inst. 2003 Nov 5; 95(21):15788–6.

Jefferson Encyclopedia: http://wiki.monticello.org/.

USDA Tomato Nutrition Stats: http://www.nal.usda.gov/fnic/foodcomp/cgi-bin/
list_nut_edit.pl

SIDEBAR CITATIONS:

Organic Tomatoes
Mitchell AE, et al.
Ten-year comparison of the influence of organic and conventional crop management practices on
the content of flavonoids in tomatoes.
J Agric Food Chem. 2007 Jul 25; 55(15):6154–9.

Tomatoes and Prostate Cancer
Etminan M, et al.
The role of tomato products and lycopene in the prevention of prostate cancer: A meta-analysis of
observational studies.
Cancer Epidemiol Biomarkers Prev. 2004 Mar; 13(3):340–5.

2 Avocados

Vartiainen E, Puska P, Pekkanen J.
Changes in risk factor explain changes in mortality from ischaemic heart disease
in Finland.
British Medical Journal, 1994; 309:23.

Puska P, Vartiainen E, Tuomilehto J, et al.
Changes in premature deaths in Finland: Successful long-term prevention of cardiovascular
diseases.
Bulletin of the World Health Organization 1998; 76(4): 419–25.

http://www.americanheart.org/presenter.jhtml?identifier=3045795.

Mitrou PN, Kipnis V, Thiébaut AC, et al.
Mediterranean dietary pattern and prediction of all-cause mortality in a US population: Results
    from the NIH-AARP Diet and Health Study.
Arch Intern Med. 2007 Dec 10; 167(22):2461–8.

Ascherio A, Katan MB, Zock PL, Stampfer MJ, Willett WC.
Trans fatty acids and coronary heart disease.
N Engl J Med. 1999 Jun 24; 340(25):1994–8.

Hu FB, Stampfer MJ, Manson JE, et al.
Dietary fat intake and the risk of coronary heart disease in women.
N Engl J Med. 1997 Nov 20; 337(21):1491–9.

Calorie totals and nutrition information for avocados based on the USDA Nutrition Database.

Nutrition information for McDonald's French fries and salad dressings courtesy of nutrition
    .mcdonalds.com.

SIDEBAR CITATIONS:

Avocado and Salad
Carotenoid absorption from salad and salsa by humans is enhanced by the addition of avocado or
    avocado oil.
Unlu NZ, Bohn T, Clinton SK, Schwartz SJ.
J Nutr. 2005 Mar; 135(3):431–6.

Avocado vs. Butter
Effects of avocado fruit puree and oatrim as fat replacers on the physical, textural and sensory
    properties of oatmeal cookies.
Wekwete B, Navder K.
J Food Qual. 2008 Mar; 31(2):131–41

3 Beets

Detopoulou P, Panagiotakos DB, et al.
Dietary choline and betaine intakes in relation to concentrations of inflammatory markers in
    healthy adults: The ATTICA study.
Am J Clin Nutr. 2008 Feb; 87(2):424–30.

Olthof MR, van Vliet T, et al.
Low dose betaine supplementation leads to immediate and long term lowering of plasma homocys-
teine in healthy men and women.
J Nutr. 2003 Dec; 133(12):4135–8.

Ilnitskii AP, Iurchenko VA.
Effect of fruit and vegetable juices on the changes in the production of carcinogenic N-nitroso
compounds in human gastric juice.
Vopr Pitan 1993 Jul–Sep; (4):44–6.

Appel LJ, Moore TJ, et al.
A clinical trial of the effects of dietary patterns on blood pressure. DASH Collaborative Research
Group.
N Engl J Med. 1997; 336:1117–24.

Webb AJ, Patel N, et al.
Acute blood pressure lowering, vasoprotective, and antiplatelet properties of dietary nitrate via
bioconversion to nitrite.
Hypertension. 2008 Mar; 51(3):784–90.

Tesoriere L, Butera D, et al.
Supplementation with cactus pear (Opuntia ficus-indica) fruit decreases oxidative stress in healthy
humans: A comparative study with vitamin C.
Am J Clin Nutr. 2004 Aug; 80(2):391–5.

Rouse IL, Beilin LJ, et al.
Blood-pressure-lowering effect of a vegetarian diet: Controlled trial in normotensive subjects.
Lancet. 1983; 1:5–10.

Hung HC, Joshipura KJ, et al.
Fruit and vegetable intake and risk of major chronic disease.
J Natl Cancer Inst. 2004; 96:1577–84.

Larsen FJ, Ekblom B, et al.
Effects of dietary nitrate on blood pressure in healthy volunteers.
N Engl J Med. 2006; 355:2792–3.

Appel LJ, Brands MW, et al.
Dietary approaches to prevent and treat hypertension: A scientific statement from the American
Heart Association.
Hypertension. 2006; 47:296–308.

Wink, DA, Paolocci N.
Mother was right: eat your vegetables and do not spit!: When oral nitrate helps with high blood
    pressure.
Hypertension 2008; 51:617–9.

SIDEBAR CITATIONS:

Velvety Beet and Leek Soup
Shimazaki Y, Shirota T, et al.
Intake of dairy products and periodontal disease: The Hisayama Study.
Periodontol. 2008 Jan; 79(1):131–7.

Baharav E, Mor F, et al.
Lactobacillus GG bacteria ameliorate arthritis in Lewis rats.
J Nutr. 2004 Aug; 134(8):1964–9.

Meydani SN, Ha WK.
Immunologic effects of yogurt.
Am J Clin Nutr. 2000 Apr; 71(4):861–72.

Is Juicing All It's Cracked Up to Be?
Dai Q, Borenstein AR, et al.
Fruit and vegetable juices and Alzheimer's disease: The Kame Project.
Am J Med. 2006 Sep; 119(9):751–9.

Percival SS, Bukowski JF, Milner J.
Bioactive food components that enhance gammadelta T cell function may play a role in cancer
    prevention.
J Nutr. 2008 Jan; 138(1):1–4.

McEligot AJ, Rock CL, et al.
Comparison of serum carotenoid responses between women consuming vegetable juice and women
    consuming raw or cooked vegetables.
Cancer Epidemiol Biomarkers Prev. 1999 Mar; 8(3):227–31.

Blanck HM, Gillespie C, et al.
Trends in fruit and vegetable consumption among U.S. men and women, 1994–2005.
Prev Chronic Dis. 2008 Apr; 5(2):A35.

Beet and Zucchini Lasagne
Allen LH, Ahluwalia N.
Improving iron status through diet. The application of knowledge concerning dietary iron bioavail-
    abiliy in human populations.
OMNI Technical Papers, No. 8. Arlington, VA: John Snow International.

Hallberg L, Brune M, Rossander L.
Effect of ascorbic acid on iron absorption from different types of meals: Studies with ascorbic-acid-
    rich foods and synthetic ascorbic acid given in different amounts with different meals.
Hum Nutr Appl Nutr. 1986 Apr; 40(2):97–113.

Teucher B, Olivares M, Cori H.
Enhancers of iron absorption: Ascorbic acid and other organic acids.
Int J Vitam Nutr Res. 2004 Nov; 74(6):403–19.

Cook JD, Reddy MB.
Effect of ascorbic acid intake on nonheme-iron absorption from a complete diet.
Am J Clin Nutr. 2001 Jan; 73(1):93–8.

Beef and Beet Stew
Eynard AR, Lopez CB.
Conjugated linoleic acid (CLA) versus saturated fats/cholesterol: Their proportion in fatty and lean
    meats may affect the risk of developing colon cancer.
Lipids Health Dis. 2003 Aug 29; 2:6.

Navarro A, Díaz MP, Muñoz SE, Lantieri MJ, Eynard AR.
Characterization of meat consumption and risk of colorectal cancer in Cordoba, Argentina.
Nutrition. 2003 Jan; 19(1):7–10.

Beauchesne-Rondeau E, Gascon A, Bergeron J, Jacques H.
Plasma lipids and lipoproteins in hypercholesterolemic men fed a lipid-lowering diet containing
    lean beef, lean fish, or poultry.
Am J Clin Nutr. 2003 Mar; 77(3):587–93.

4 Spinach

Freedman ND, Park Y, et al.
Fruit and vegetable intake and esophageal cancer in a large prospective cohort study.
Int J Cancer. 2007 Dec 15; 121(12):2753–60.

Rai A, Mohapatra SC, Shukla HS.
Correlates between vegetable consumption and gallbladder cancer.
Eur J Cancer Prev. 2006 Apr; 15(2):134–7.

Jian L, Du CJ, et al.
Do dietary lycopene and other carotenoids protect against prostate cancer?
Int J Cancer. 2005 Mar 1; 113(6):1010–4.

Slattery ML, Benson J, et al.
Carotenoids and colon cancer.
Am J Clin Nutr. 2000 Feb; 71(2):575–82.

Longnecker MP, Newcomb PA, et al.
Intake of carrots, spinach, and supplements containing vitamin A in relation to risk of breast
    cancer.
Cancer Epidemiol Biomarkers Prev. 1997 Nov; 6(11):887–92.

Casagrande SS, Wang Y, et al.
Have Americans increased their fruit and vegetable intake? The trends between 1988 and 2002.
Am J Prev Med. 2007 Apr; 32(4):257–63.

Guenther PM, Dodd KW, et al.
Most Americans eat much less than recommended amounts of fruits and vegetables.
J Am Diet Assoc. 2006 Sep; 106(9):1371–9.

Mortality data from CDC/National Center for Health Statistics:
http://www.cdc.gov/nchs/FASTATS/deaths.htm.

USDA ORAC scores accessed at: http://www.ars.usda.gov/Services/docs.htm?docid=15866.

SIDEBAR CITATIONS:

Spinach and Lamb over Spinach Farfalle
Associations of vegetable and fruit consumption with age-related cognitive change.
Morris MC, Evans DA, Tangney CC, Bienias JL, Wilson RS.
Neurology. 2006 Oct 24; 67(8):1370–6.

Getting Kids to Eat Spinach
The persistence of false beliefs.
Laney C, Fowler NB, Nelson KJ, Bernstein DM, Loftus EF.
Acta Psychol (Amst). 2008 Sep; 129(1):190–7.

5 Quinoa

Schlick G, Bubenheim DL.
Quinoa: An emerging new crop with potential for CELSS.
NASA Technical Paper 3422. November 1993.

Nutrition content for quinoa accessed from USDA, available at: http://www.nal.usda.gov/fnic
/foodcomp/search/.

Mozaffarian D, Kamineni A, et al.
Lifestyle risk factors and new-onset diabetes mellitus in older adults: The cardiovascular health
study.
Arch Intern Med. 2009 Apr 27; 169(8):798–807.

Rimm EB, Ascherio A, et al.
Vegetable, fruit, and cereal fiber intake and risk of coronary heart disease among men.
JAMA. 1996 Feb 14; 275(6):447–51.

Berti C, Riso P, et al.
Effect on appetite control of minor cereal and pseudocereal products.
Br J Nutr. 2005 Nov; 94(5):850 8.

Barclay AW, Petocz P, et al.
Glycemic index, glycemic load, and chronic disease risk: A meta-analysis of observational studies.
Am J Clin Nutr. 2008 Mar; 87(3):627–37. Review.

Nilsson AC, Ostman EM, et al.
Effect of cereal test breakfasts differing in glycemic index and content of indigestible carbohydrates
on daylong glucose tolerance in healthy subjects.
Am J Clin Nutr. 2008 Mar; 87(3):645–54.

SIDEBAR CITATIONS:

Cinnamon
Oxygen radical absorbance capacity (ORAC) of selected foods—2007.
Nutrient Data Laboratory, USDA.

Hlebowicz J, Darwiche G, et al.
Effect of cinnamon on postprandial blood glucose, gastric emptying, and satiety in healthy subjects.
Am J Clin Nutr. 2007 Jun; 85(6):1552–6.

Hlebowicz J, Hlebowicz A, et al.

Effects of 1 and 3 g cinnamon on gastric emptying, satiety, and postprandial blood glucose, insulin, glucose-dependent insulinotropic polypeptide, glucagon-like peptide 1, and ghrelin concentrations in healthy subjects.

Am J Clin Nutr. 2009 Mar; 89(3):815–21.

Quinoa and Life Expectancy
Pereira MA, O'Reilly E, et al.
Dietary fiber and risk of coronary heart disease: A pooled analysis of cohort studies.
Arch Intern Med. 2004 Feb 23; 164(4):370–6.

6 Lentils

Nicklas TA, Farris RP, et al.
Dietary fiber intake of children and young adults: The Bogalusa Heart Study.

J Am Diet Assoc. 1995 Feb; 95(2):209–14.
National Fiber Council Survey: http://www.nationalfibercouncil.org/pdfs/Lead_Release.pdf.

Lustig RH.
The "skinny" on childhood obesity: How our western environment starves kids' brains.
Pediatr Ann. 2006 Dec; 35(12):898–902, 905–7. Review.

Nutrition content for lentils accessed from USDA, available at: http://www.nal.usda.gov/fnic/foodcomp/search/.

Anderson JW, Baird P, et al.
Health benefits of dietary fiber.
Nutr Rev. 2009 Apr; 67(4):188–205.

Estruch R, Martinez-Gonzalez MA, et al.
Effects of dietary fiber intake on risk factors for cardiovascular disease in subjects at high risk.
J Epidemiol Community Health. Epub 2009 Mar 15.

Hamedani A, Akhavan T, et al.
Reduced energy intake at breakfast is not compensated for at lunch if a high-insoluble-fiber cereal replaces a low-fiber cereal.
Am J Clin Nutr. 2009 May; 89(5):1343–9. Epub 2009 Apr 1.

Aller R, de Luis DA, et al.

Effect of soluble fiber intake in lipid and glucose levels in healthy subjects: A randomized clinical trial.

Diabetes Res Clin Pract. 2004 Jul; 65(1):7–11.

Sinha R, Cross AJ, et al.

Meat intake and mortality: A prospective study of over half a million people.

Arch Intern Med. 2009 Mar 23; 169(6):562–71.

SIDEBAR CITATIONS:

Turmeric

Goel A, Kunnumakkara AB, et al.

Curcumin as "curecumin": from kitchen to clinic.

Biochem Pharmacol. 2008 Feb 15; 75(4):787–809. Epub 2007 Aug 19. Review.

Jagetia GC, Aggarwal BB.

"Spicing up" of the immune system by curcumin.

J Clin Immunol. 2007 Jan; 27(1):19–35. Epub 2007 Jan 9. Review.

Lentils and Glycemic Index

Foster-Powell K, Holt SH, et al.

International table of glycemic index and glycemic load values: 2002.

Am J Clin Nutr. 2002 Jul; 76(1):5–56.

http://www.glycemicindex.com/.

The Better Burger

Ralof, J.

AAAS: Climate-friendly dining . . . meats

http://www.sciencenews.org. February 2009.

7 Cabbage

Ju YH, Carlson KE, et al.

Estrogenic effects of extracts from cabbage, fermented cabbage, and acidified brussels sprouts on growth and gene expression of estrogen-dependent human breast cancer (MCF-7) cells.

J Agric Food Chem. 2000 Oct; 48(10):4628–34.

Pathak DR, et al.
Joint association of high cabbage/sauerkraut intake at 12–13 years of age and adulthood associated with reduced breast cancer risk in Polish migrant women.
Abstract number 3697. Presented at the AACR 4th Annual Conference on Frontiers in Cancer Prevention Research, Baltimore, Maryland. 2005.

Cornblatt BS, Ye L, et al.
Preclinical and clinical evaluation of sulforaphane for chemoprevention in the breast.
Carcinogenesis. 2007 Jul; 28(7):1485–90.

Fahey JW, Zhang Y, et al.
Broccoli sprouts: An exceptionally rich source of inducers of enzymes that protect against chemical carcinogens.
Proc Natl Acad Sci U S A. 1997 Sep 16; 94(19):10367–72.

Hanf V, Gonder U.
Nutrition and primary prevention of breast cancer: Foods, nutrients and breast cancer risk.
Eur J Obstet Gynecol Reprod Biol. 2005 Dec 1; 123(2):139–49.

Palmer S.
Diet, nutrition, and cancer.
Prog Food Nutr Sci. 1985; 9(3–4):283–341.

Zhang Y, Talalay P, et al.
A major inducer of anticarcinogenic protective enzymes from broccoli: Isolation and elucidation of structure.
Proc Natl Acad Sci U S A. 1992 Mar 15; 89(6):2399–403.

Bradlow HL.
Indole-3-carbinol as a chemoprotective agent in breast and prostate cancer.
In Vivo. 2008 Jul–Aug; 22(4):441–5. Review.

Nutritional content for cruciferous vegetables accessed from USDA, at: http://www.nal.usda.gov/fnic/foodcomp/search/.

SIDEBAR CITATIONS:

Cabbage vs. Broccoli
Somerset SM, Johannot L.
Dietary flavonoid sources in Australian adults.
Nutr Cancer. 2008; 60(4):442–9.

Huxley RR, Neil HA.
The relation between dietary flavonol intake and coronary heart disease mortality: A meta-analysis of prospective cohort studies.
Eur J Clin Nutr. 2003 Aug; 57(8):904–8.

Huxley RR, Hawkins MH, et al.
Risk of fatal stroke in patients with treated familial hypercholesterolemia: A prospective registry study.
Stroke. 2003 Jan; 34(1):22–5.

8 *Super Fish*

Broadhurst CL, Cunnane SC, et al.
Rift Valley lake fish and shellfish provided brain-specific nutrition for early Homo.
British Journal of Nutrition. 1998; (79)3–21.

Stringer CB, Finlayson JC, et al.
Neanderthal exploitation of marine mammals in Gibraltar.
Proc Natl Acad Sci U S A. 2008 Sep 23; 105(38):14319–24.

Barberger-Gateau P, Raffaitin C, et al.
Dietary patterns and risk of dementia: The Three-City cohort study.
Neurology. 2007 Nov 13; 69(20):1921–30.

Mozaffarian D, Longstreth WT Jr, et al.
Fish consumption and stroke risk in elderly individuals: The cardiovascular health study.
Arch Intern Med. 2005 Jan 24; 165(2):200–6.

He K, Rimm EB, Merchant A, et al.
Fish consumption and risk of stroke in men.
JAMA. 2002 Dec 25; 288(24):3130–6.

Albert CM, Hennekens CH, et al.
Fish consumption and risk of sudden cardiac death.
JAMA. 1998 Jan 7; 279(1):23–8.

Hu FB, Bronner L, Willett WC, et al.
Fish and omega-3 fatty acid intake and risk of coronary heart disease in women.
JAMA. 2002 Apr 10; 287(14):1815–21.

Weber HS, Selimi D, Huber G.
Prevention of cardiovascular diseases and highly concentrated n-3 polyunsaturated fatty acids
     (PUFAs).
Herz. 2006 Dec; 31 Suppl 3:24–30. Review.

McLaughlin J, Middaugh J, et al.
Adipose tissue triglyceride fatty acids and atherosclerosis in Alaska Natives and non-Natives.
Atherosclerosis. 2005 Aug; 181(2):353–62.

Newman WP, Middaugh JP, et al.
Atherosclerosis in Alaska Natives and non-natives.
Lancet. 1993 Apr 24; 341(8852):1056–7.

Yamagishi K, Iso H, et al.
Fish, omega-3 polyunsaturated fatty acids, and mortality from cardiovascular diseases in a nation-
     wide community-based cohort of Japanese men and women. The JACC (Japan Collaborative
     Cohort Study for Evaluation of Cancer Risk) Study.
J Am Coll Cardiol. 2008 Sep 16; 52(12):988–96.

Iso H, Kobayashi M, et al.
Intake of fish and n3 fatty acids and risk of coronary heart disease among Japanese: The Japan
     Public Health Center-Based (JPHC) Study Cohort I.
Circulation. 2006 Jan 17; 113(2):195–202.

Calò L, Bianconi L, et al.
N-3 fatty acids for the prevention of atrial fibrillation after coronary artery bypass surgery: A ran-
     domized, controlled trial.
J Am Coll Cardiol. 2005 May 17; 45(10):1723–8.

Oh RC, Beresford SA, et al.
The fish in secondary prevention of heart disease (FISH) survey: Primary care physicians and
     omega 3 fatty acid prescribing behaviors.
J Am Board Fam Med. 2006 Sep–Oct; 19(5):459–67.

Rosenthal, Libby.
In Europe it's fish oil after heart attacks, but not in U.S.
The New York Times, October 2006.

SIDEBAR CITATIONS:

Mercury Be Gone!
Passos CJ, Mergler D, et al.
Eating tropical fruit reduces mercury exposure from fish consumption in the Brazilian Amazon.
Environ Res. 2003 Oct; 93(2):123–30.

Passos CJ, Mergler D, et al.
Epidemiologic confirmation that fruit consumption influences mercury exposure in riparian communities in the Brazilian Amazon.
Environ Res. 2007 Oct; 105(2):183–93.

http://docs.lib.purdue.edu/dissertations/AAI3210789/.

Surf 'n' Turf
Zhang J, Svehlíková V, et al.
Synergy between sulforaphane and selenium in the induction of thioredoxin reductase 1 requires both transcriptional and translational modulation.
Carcinogenesis. 2003 Mar; 24(3):497–503.

Brain Food
Oken E, Østerdal ML, et al.
Associations of maternal fish intake during pregnancy and breastfeeding duration with attainment of developmental milestones in early childhood: A study from the Danish National Birth Cohort.
Am J Clin Nutr. 2008 Sep; 88(3):789–96.

Oken E, Radesky JS, et al.
Maternal fish intake during pregnancy, blood mercury levels, and child cognition at age 3 years in a US cohort.
Am J Epidemiol. 2008 May 15; 167(10):1171–81.

Marinade Magic
Sinha R, Chow WH, et al.
Well-done, grilled red meat increases the risk of colorectal adenomas.
Cancer Res. 1999 Sep 1; 59(17):4320–4.

Stolzenberg-Solomon RZ, Cross AJ, et al.
Meat and meat-mutagen intake and pancreatic cancer risk in the NIH-AARP cohort.
Cancer Epidemiol Biomarkers Prev. 2007 Dec; 16(12):2664–75.

Steck SE, Gaudet MM, et al.
Cooked meat and risk of breast cancer: Lifetime versus recent dietary intake.
Epidemiology. 2007 May; 18(3):373–82.

Sinha R, Rothman N.
Role of well-done, grilled red meat, heterocyclic amines (HCAs) in the etiology of human cancer.
Cancer Lett. 1999 Sep 1; 143(2):189–94.

9 Nuts

Strait DS, Weber GW, et al.
The feeding biomechanics and dietary ecology of Australopithecus africanus.
Proc Natl Acad Sci U S A. 2009 Feb 17; 106 (7):2124–9.

Kelly JH Jr, Sabaté J.
Nuts and coronary heart disease: An epidemiological perspective.
Br J Nutr. 2006 Nov; 96 Suppl 2:S61–7.

Blomhoff R, Carlsen MH, et al.
Health benefits of nuts: Potential role of antioxidants.
Br J Nutr. 2006 Nov; 96 Suppl 2:S52–60.

Nutritional content for various nuts found at: http://www.nal.usda.gov/fnic/foodcomp/search/.

Bes-Rastrollo M, Sabaté J, et al.
Nut consumption and weight gain in a Mediterranean cohort: The SUN study.
Obesity (Silver Spring). 2007 Jan; 15(1):107–16.

Hollis J, Mattes R.
Effect of chronic consumption of almonds on body weight in healthy humans.
Br J Nutr. 2007 Sep; 98(3):651–6.

Wien MA, Sabaté JM, et al.
Almonds vs complex carbohydrates in a weight reduction program.
Int J Obes Relat Metab Disord. 2003 Nov; 27(11):1365–72.

SIDEBAR CITATIONS:

Peanut Salad
Yeh CC, You SL, et al.
Peanut consumption and reduced risk of colorectal cancer in women: A prospective study in
     Taiwan. World J Gastroenterol. 2006 Jan 14; 12(2):222–7.

Broiled Lamb Chops with Walnut and Mint *Gremolata* / Walnuts and Sleep
Reiter RJ, Manchester LC, Tan DX.
Melatonin in walnuts: Influence on levels of melatonin and total antioxidant capacity of blood.
Nutrition. 2005 Sep; 21(9):920–4.

10 Berries

Kuskoski EM, Asuero AG, et al.
Wild fruits and pulps of frozen fruits: Antioxidant activity, polyphenols and anthocyanins
Cienc Rural. 2006 July–Aug; 36(4).

Halvorsen BL, Carlsen MH, et al.
Content of redox-active compounds (ie, antioxidants) in foods consumed in the United States.
Am J Clin Nutr. 2006 Jul; 84(1):95–135.

Hager TJ, Howard LR, et al.
Ellagitannin composition of blackberry as determined by HPLC-ESI-MS and MALDI-TOF-MS.
J Agric Food Chem. 2008 Feb 13; 56(3):661–9. Epub 2008 Jan 23.

Oxygen Radical Absorbance Capacity of Selected Foods.
Nutrient Data Laboratory, Agricultural Research Service, United States Department of Agricul-
     ture, November 2007.

Food and Nutrition Board, Institute of Medicine.
Dietary Reference Intakes for Water, Potassium, Sodium, Chloride, and Sulfate.
Washington, DC: National Academies Press, 2004:173–246.

Hopkins Tanne J.
Americans are told to reduce sodium and increase potassium intake.
BMJ. 2004 Feb 28; 328(7438):485.

Nutrient data for berries available from the USDA at: http://www.nal.usda.gov/fnic/foodcomp/search/.

SIDEBAR CITATIONS:

What Berries Might Do for You: A Scientific Breakdown
Erlund I, et al.
Favorable effects of berry consumption on platelet function, blood pressure, and HDL cholesterol.
Am J Clin Nutr. 2008 Feb; 87(2):323–31.

Getting forgetful? Then blueberries may hold the key.
The Peninsula College of Medicine and Dentistry.
ScienceDaily. April 12, 2008.

Stoner G, et al.
Regression of rectal polyps in familial adenomatous polyposis patients with freeze-dried black
    raspberries.
Cancer Prev Res 2008; 1(7 Suppl):PR-14.

Giovannucci E, Ascherio A, et al.
Intake of carotenoids and retinol in relation to risk of prostate cancer.
J Natl Cancer Inst. 1995 Dec 6; 87(23):1767–76.

Ricotta Rocks!
Hoffman JR, Falvo MJ.
Protein–Which is best?
Journal of Sports Science and Medicine. 2004; 3:118–30.

Blueberries as Bacteria Killer?
Ofek I, Goldhar J, Sharon N.
Anti-Escherichia coli adhesin activity of cranberry and blueberry juices.
Adv Exp Med Biol. 1996; 408:179–83. Review.

Balsamic Berry Salad
Cho E, Seddon JM, et al.
Prospective study of intake of fruits, vegetables, vitamins, and carotenoids and risk of age-related
    maculopathy.
Arch Ophthalmol. 2004 Jun; 122(6):883–92.

INDEX

Zucchini-Layered Salmon with Stewed Eggplant, 186–87